Contents

Summary

In 2012, the Department of Defense (DoD) spent $52 billion on health care for service members, retirees, and their families. The department offers health care to nearly 10 million people through its TRICARE program, an integrated system of military health care providers and regional networks of civilian providers. Established in 1993, TRICARE now consists of three major plans: TRICARE Prime, TRICARE Standard, and TRICARE Extra. The following groups of people are eligible to participate in TRICARE (with the respective populations in 2012 shown in parentheses):

- All members of the four military branches as well as members of the Coast Guard and the commissioned corps of the Public Health Service and of the National Oceanic and Atmospheric Administration (1.8 million);

- Families of current service members (2.6 million); and

- Retired service members and their families (5.2 million).

The cost of providing that care has increased rapidly as a share of the defense budget over the past decade, outpacing growth in the economy, growth in per capita health care spending in the United States, and growth in funding for DoD's base budget (which finances the department's routine activities but has excluded funding for operations in Iraq and Afghanistan). Between 2000 and 2012, funding for military health care increased by 130 percent, over and above the effects of overall inflation in the economy. In 2000, funding for health care accounted for about 6 percent of DoD's base budget; by 2012, that share had reached nearly 10 percent. By 2028, health care would claim 11 percent of the cost of implementing DoD's plans, the Congressional Budget Office (CBO) estimates (see Summary Figure 1).

The Budget Control Act of 2011 (as modified by subsequent legislation) capped funding for national defense between 2014 and 2021 at about 10 percent below CBO's projection of the cost of DoD's plans as of November 2013, using DoD's estimates of prices.[1] The share of health care costs in future budgets will depend on how DoD adjusts its plans to comply with those caps. For example, if the growth in health care costs is unconstrained by new policies and cuts are made in funding for other defense activities (such as the development and procurement of weapon systems), then health care costs could account for an even larger percentage of the department's future spending.

What Have Been the Primary Causes of Growth in Spending for Military Health Care?

The rapid increases in the cost of military health care are often attributed to the following factors:

- *New and expanded TRICARE benefits.* Lawmakers have expanded the TRICARE benefit in various ways. TRICARE for Life, a new benefit established in 2002, eliminates most of the out-of-pocket costs faced by Medicare-eligible military retirees and their families. Other expanded benefits provide coverage to members of the National Guard and Reserves when they are not serving on active duty.

---

1. For CBO's projection of the overall defense budget, see Congressional Budget Office, *Long-Term Implications of the 2014 Future Years Defense Program* (November 2013), www.cbo.gov/publication/44683. The Bipartisan Budget Act of 2013, which was enacted shortly before this report was released, will have only a small effect on the cumulative limit on defense funding from 2014 through 2021.

Summary Figure 1.

Actual and Projected Costs for Military Health Care as a Share of DoD's Base Budget, 1990 to 2028

(Percent)

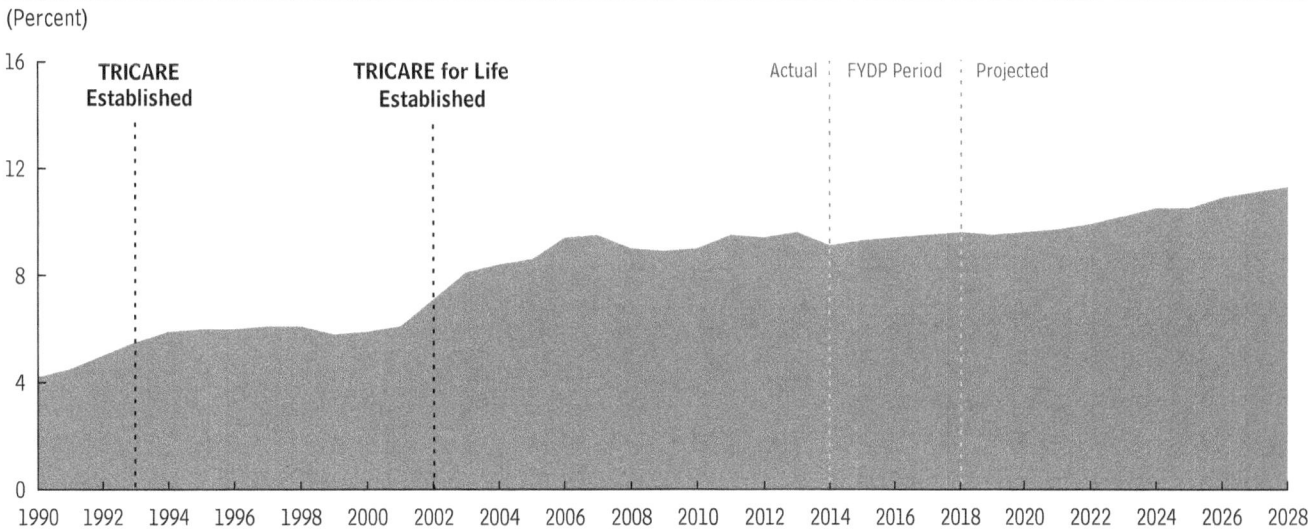

Source: Congressional Budget Office, *Long-Term Implications of the Fiscal Year 2014 Future Years Defense Program* (November 2013), www.cbo.gov/publication/44683.

Notes: In this figure, the FYDP projection spans the five-year period from 2014 through 2018. CBO's projection spans the years 2019 through 2028.

The historical data for military health care include supplemental and emergency funding for overseas contingency operations through 2013, but those funds are not included in CBO's projections.

DoD = Department of Defense; FYDP = Future Years Defense Program.

■ *Increased utilization fostered by financial incentives to use TRICARE.* The share of health care costs that TRICARE users pay is much lower than the costs paid by most civilian consumers who use private or employment-based health insurance. Depending on which plan people select, the cost of TRICARE may include enrollment fees (which are charged annually and are similar to health insurance premiums in the civilian market), copayments (which are fees charged each time medical care is accessed), and deductibles (which are the amounts that users must pay before TRICARE will pay a claim). TRICARE's comparatively low out-of-pocket costs have had two effects: First, the number of users has increased as people switched from more expensive plans to TRICARE; and second, TRICARE participants have increased the volume of health services they consume. (The total number of people enrolled in TRICARE Prime—the most costly plan to DoD—rose by 8 percent between 2003 and 2012. And DoD estimates that, in 2012, the average person enrolled in TRICARE Prime used 50 percent more outpatient

services than a civilian of comparable age participating in a health maintenance organization.)

■ *Medical costs of recent wars.* Although DoD has received supplemental funding for combat-related medical care, that funding has been relatively small and should decrease as operations end and as service members who participated in those operations separate from the military and transition to other sources of health care, including the Veterans Health Administration.

CBO finds that the first two factors explain most of the growth in military health care costs since 2000; the third has had a comparatively small effect on DoD's spending.

What Are Some Approaches to Controlling Costs?

DoD's total budget will be constrained through 2021 by caps on funding for national defense that were established under the Budget Control Act of 2011 (and modified by the American Taxpayer Relief Act of 2012 and the

Bipartisan Budget Act of 2013). In a fiscal climate in which the department's overall budget can increase only slowly, continued rapid growth in military health care costs could force DoD to reduce spending in other areas, such as force structure, military readiness, and weapons modernization.

Policymakers have considered various initiatives to slow federal spending for health care in general, some of which could apply to DoD. CBO examined three:

■ Better management of chronic diseases,

■ More effective administration of the military health care system, and

■ Increased cost sharing for retirees who use TRICARE.

In CBO's judgment, only the last of those approaches has the potential to generate significant savings for DoD. The other two could generate modest savings, but they would not address the primary drivers of health care costs for DoD.

Better Management of Chronic Diseases

Disease management programs aim to reduce costly emergency room visits and hospitalizations by better monitoring and controlling patients' symptoms before they become acute. Although disease management programs have the potential to improve health outcomes, DoD's experience to date suggests that savings from such programs would probably be relatively small, perhaps several tens of millions of dollars each year.

More Effective Administration of the Military Health Care System

CBO explored two such approaches: close DoD's medical school, the Uniformed Services University of the Health Sciences (USUHS), while expanding the number of scholarships provided to students attending civilian medical schools; and hire more auditors to reduce fraud. Substituting scholarships for tuition-free medical education at USUHS would reduce costs but by only a small amount because the school itself is small. Reducing fraud by increasing the number of auditors is intuitively appealing, but DoD's Office of Program Integrity is small, so even doubling its size would result in relatively little savings.

The savings realized from either of those measures would range from a few million dollars to about $150 million a year, significantly less than the savings that would result from cost-sharing options.

Increased Cost Sharing for Retirees Who Use TRICARE

CBO analyzed three options for increasing the share of health care costs borne by users of TRICARE:

■ *Option 1:* Increase medical cost sharing for beneficiaries who have already retired from the military but who are not yet eligible for Medicare (sometimes called working-age retirees, they are generally between the ages of 40 and 65).

■ *Option 2:* Make working-age retirees and their families ineligible for TRICARE Prime, the most costly program for DoD, but allow them to continue using other TRICARE plans after paying an annual fee.[2]

■ *Option 3:* Introduce minimum out-of-pocket requirements for Medicare-eligible retirees and their family members (generally those over 65 years of age) to access TRICARE for Life.

Assessing the budgetary effects of the options is complicated because each option could affect the behavior of current TRICARE beneficiaries. For example, higher out-of-pocket costs for TRICARE would cause some current users to switch to other forms of health insurance. If they switched to other federal plans (such as that offered by the Veterans Health Administration), spending for those plans would increase. If they switched to health insurance provided by their current employer, a greater share of their compensation would become nontaxable, reducing federal tax revenues.

The reduction in the federal deficit from these options over the next 10 years, including effects on spending by DoD and the other uniformed services, the Department of Veterans Affairs, Medicare, the Federal Employees Health Benefits program, and Medicaid, would range from roughly $20 billion to $60 billion, if lawmakers reduced total appropriations accordingly (see the first three columns in Summary Table 1). The full effects on the federal budget are shown in Chapter 2.

---

2. TRICARE Prime is modeled on civilian health maintenance organizations and, unlike most of TRICARE's other plans, requires beneficiaries to enroll every year. Compared with other TRICARE plans, TRICARE Prime offers beneficiaries the lowest out-of-pocket costs but entails the highest per-user costs for DoD.

Summary Table 1.

Cumulative Budgetary Effects of Policy Options That Would Raise Military Retirees' Cost Sharing, 2015 to 2023

(Billions of dollars)

	Change in the Federal Budget			Change in DoD's Budget Authority
	Discretionary Outlays	Mandatory Outlays	Revenues	
Option 1: Increase Medical Cost Sharing for Military Retirees Who Are Not Yet Eligible for Medicare	-19.7	-0.3	-1.6	-24.1
Option 2: Make Military Retirees Ineligible for TRICARE Prime; Allow Continued Use of Standard and Extra With an Annual Fee	-71.0	0.5	-10.5	-89.6
Option 3: Introduce Minimum Out-of-Pocket Requirements for TRICARE for Life	0	-30.7	0	-18.4

Source: Congressional Budget Office.

Notes: The potential spending reductions from these policy options may not be additive; implementing one option could affect the spending in another. These estimates reflect the assumption that each change would go into effect at the beginning of fiscal year 2015.

Budget authority is authority provided by law to enter into obligations that will result in outlays of federal funds. Outlays are payments made to liquidate obligations.

Negative numbers represent reductions in outlays or budget authority or a loss of revenues.

DoD = Department of Defense.

The estimated reductions for the three options may not be additive, however. In particular, if Option 2 was implemented and working-age retirees were prohibited from enrolling in TRICARE Prime, Option 1—allowing those enrollments but at a higher fee—would be precluded. In addition, the size of the savings would depend on the way in which the new fees were implemented. These estimates reflect the assumption that the options would be fully implemented in 2015. If the new measures were phased in more slowly, or if exemptions were provided for retirees in poor health or for those with lower earnings, the estimated spending reductions would be smaller.

Putting aside the effects on other agencies, the effect of those options on DoD alone would be different (see the fourth column in Summary Table 1). Option 2, which would eliminate the TRICARE Prime benefit for all military retirees and their families, would have the largest effect, reducing DoD's funding for health care by about $90 billion (or 17 percent) over the 2015–2023 period, CBO estimates. Implementing either Option 1 or Option 3 would lower DoD's budget for military health care by $24 billion (or 5 percent) and $18 billion (or 3 percent), respectively, from 2015 through 2023.

Those options could discourage some people from using health care services, and some patients could have adverse health outcomes if the higher costs caused them to delay seeking care. Moreover, some military retirees argue that they initially joined the military and remained for their entire careers with the understanding that they would receive medical care for free or at a very low cost after retiring. Significantly limiting TRICARE coverage for military retirees and their dependents would impose a financial cost on many of those beneficiaries and could adversely affect military retention. Some observers note, however, that the current system favors only a small fraction of military retirees because most people who join the military do not serve an entire career and will never qualify for retiree medical care through TRICARE. They argue that military health care benefits were originally intended to supplement, and not replace, benefits offered by civilian employers or by Medicare once service members retired.

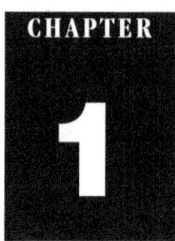

CHAPTER 1

Funding for Military Health Care

The Department of Defense (DoD) provides medical care, dental care, and prescription drug coverage to service members, retirees, and their eligible family members through the program known as TRICARE.[1] It also finances related administrative functions and ancillary activities such as those conducted at medical command headquarters, the education and training of medical personnel, medical research, and veterinary services (including the care of working animals and ensuring food safety). The cost of providing that care has increased rapidly as a share of the defense budget since 2000. Much of that increase is attributable to new and expanded TRICARE benefits and to financial incentives for people to use those benefits.

In 2012, about 8 million of nearly 10 million eligible people received health care through TRICARE.[2] Managing, supporting, and providing health care services that year required about 85,000 military personnel and 65,000 federal civilian personnel, supplemented by numerous contractors (although their numbers are not readily available). In total, DoD spent $52 billion in 2012 for health care. The Congressional Budget Office (CBO) projects that, in the absence of significant changes, spending for the military health system will continue to increase as a share of the defense budget.

---

1. TRICARE, which is funded and managed by DoD, is available to members of all seven branches of the uniformed services: the Army, Navy, Marine Corps, Air Force, Coast Guard, and the commissioned corps of the Public Health Service and of the National Oceanic and Atmospheric Administration. The first four branches represent about 97 percent of the personnel in the uniformed services.

2. Department of Defense, *Evaluation of the Tricare Program—Access, Cost and Quality: Fiscal Year 2013 Report to Congress* (February 2013), p. 15, http://go.usa.gov/jX9H. The other 2 million people are not tracked by DoD and receive health care from other sources.

The 2012 Budget for Military Health Care

Annual funding for military health care can be divided into two major components:

■ The *Defense Health Program (DHP).* The annual defense appropriation act, under the heading Defense Health Program, provides funding to the DHP for health-related operation and maintenance (O&M); procurement; and research, development, test, and evaluation (RDT&E). Most of the resources appropriated for military health care are allocated to the DHP.

■ *Military personnel.* That appropriation act, under the section called Military Personnel, also includes funding for the pay and benefits of uniformed personnel who work in the health care system, and for accrual payments on behalf of all military personnel to fund military health care for those who retire and become eligible for Medicare.

In addition to those two major categories, funding for the construction or replacement of military hospitals, clinics, or other facilities is provided in the annual military construction and veterans affairs appropriation act.

The $52 billion allocated for defense health care in 2012 was provided as follows:

■ $32.3 billion for the DHP (see Figure 1-1). Of that total, more than 90 percent ($30.4 billion) was for O&M, which funds the salaries and benefits of the civilian personnel who work in military medicine, various contracts, purchases of medical supplies, and other goods and services. The DHP also received appropriations of $1.3 billion for medical RDT&E and $600 million for procurement.

■ $1.1 billion for health-related military construction.

Figure 1-1.

Funding for Military Health Care, 2012

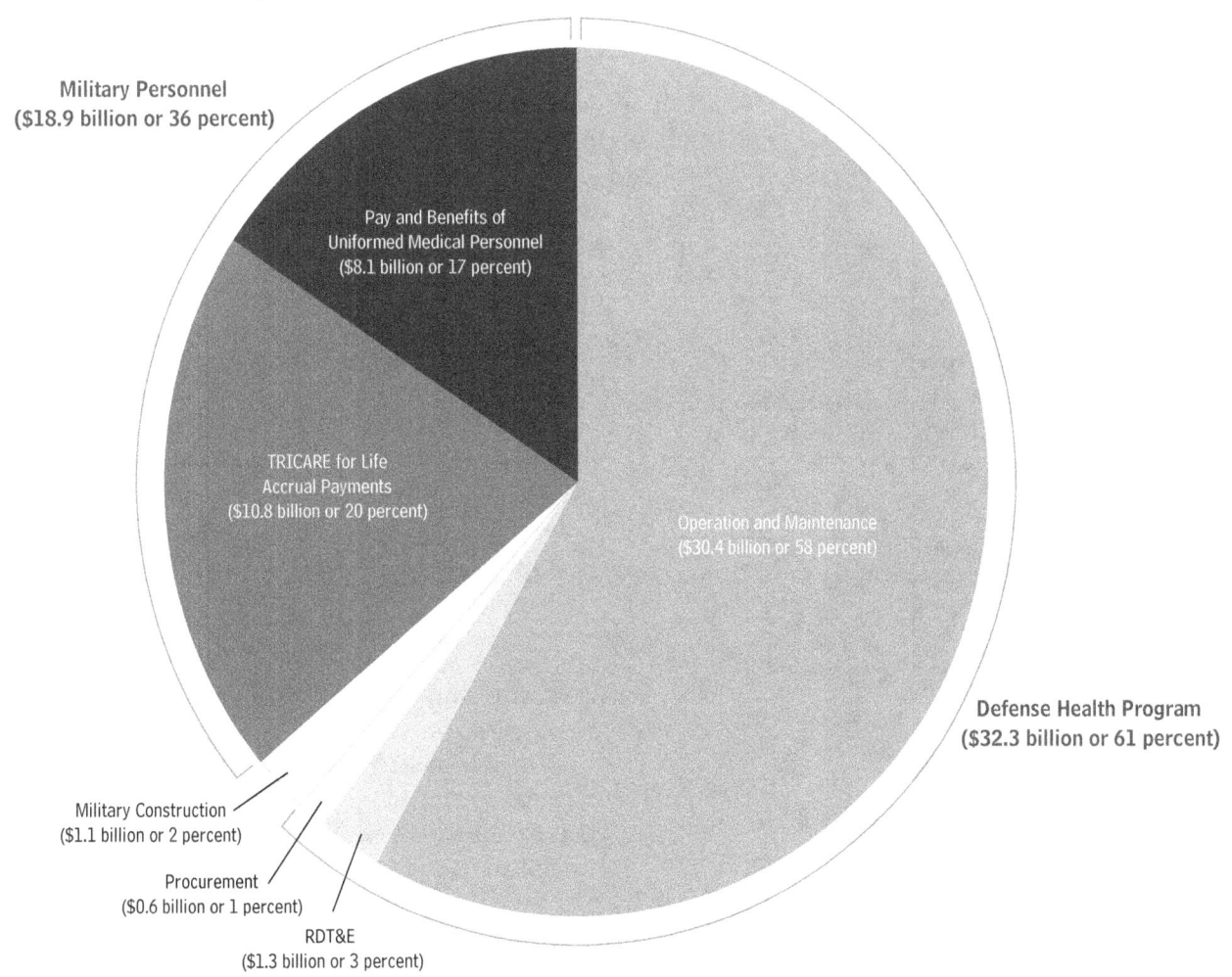

Source: Congressional Budget Office.

Notes: Annual funding for military health care can be divided into two major components. The first, called the Defense Health Program,
        includes funding for health-related operation and maintenance; procurement; and RDT&E. The second component, Military Personnel,
        includes funding for the pay and benefits of uniformed personnel who work in the health care system and for accrual payments made
        on behalf of all military personnel to the Medicare-Eligible Retiree Health Care Fund (which finances the TRICARE for Life benefit for
        those qualified personnel who retire and become eligible for Medicare). In addition to those two major categories, funding for the
        construction or replacement of military hospitals, clinics, or other facilities is provided under the "Department of Defense" section of
        the annual appropriation act for military construction and veterans affairs and related agencies.

        RDT&E = research, development, test, and evaluation.

■ $8.1 billion for pay and benefits for uniformed
  personnel working in military medicine (17 percent of
  the defense health care budget).

■ $10.8 billion for payments made to the health benefit
  program established for Medicare-eligible retirees,
  called TRICARE for Life (TFL). Those payments,
  referred to as accrual payments, represent the value of

the anticipated stream of future health care costs for
such retirees. They take into account the expected
future growth of health care costs and are made to a
special fund called the Medicare-Eligible Retiree
Health Care Fund (MERHCF). Those payments,
which are made from the Military Personnel account,
amounted to about 20 percent of funding for defense
health care.[3]

Because the appropriations for O&M and military personnel represent about 94 percent of DoD's health care funding, this report focuses on those areas and does not address activities related to RDT&E, procurement, and military construction. Also excluded is funding allocated directly to the Departments of the Army, Navy, and Air Force for providing medical care in combat areas, such as battle-aid stations and hospital ships. (Funding for most war-related military health care has generally been provided through supplemental appropriations and is discussed later in this chapter.)

TRICARE's Health Plans

Most participants in the program receive their health care through one of three major plans—TRICARE Prime, TRICARE Standard, or TRICARE Extra:

■ *TRICARE Prime* is a managed care option similar to that provided by a health maintenance organization (HMO). Of the 8.1 million people who used the TRICARE benefit in 2012, about two-thirds (5.5 million) were enrolled in Prime. Like civilian HMOs, the plan features a primary care manager (either a military or civilian health care provider) who oversees care and provides referrals to visit specialists. To ensure their health and physical readiness, active-duty service members are required to use Prime. They pay no annual enrollment fee or premium for the coverage, nor do they incur other out-of-pocket expenses, such as copayments and deductibles, for the medical care they receive. Their family members must enroll annually—also at no cost—if they wish to participate in the plan. Retired military members and their families who are not yet eligible for Medicare (generally those under the age of 65) may also enroll, but they are charged an annual enrollment fee (similar to an annual premium).

■ *TRICARE Standard* is a fee-for-service option that does not require beneficiaries to enroll in order to participate. Compared with TRICARE Prime, the Standard plan allows participants greater freedom to select providers and to access care, but it also requires users to pay higher out-of-pocket costs. In addition to satisfying an annual deductible, beneficiaries who use the Standard option must pay any difference between a provider's billed charges and the rate of reimbursement allowed under the plan.

■ *TRICARE Extra*, a variant of the Standard plan that also has no formal enrollment requirement, mirrors a civilian preferred provider organization. Under such an arrangement, network providers accept a reduced payment from TRICARE in return for the business that the local military facility refers to them, and the providers agree to file all claims for participants. In return for staying in-network, the beneficiaries' out-of-pocket costs are lower for Extra than they are for Standard.

Beneficiaries can get care under TRICARE Standard, TRICARE Extra, or both. (In this report, the term "beneficiaries" means those people that DoD identifies as being eligible to use TRICARE; "users" are those beneficiaries who enroll in or opt to use the system.) When users choose an out-of-network provider for a given medical service, they are covered under the Standard plan; if they choose an in-network provider for a different medical encounter (even within the same year), they are covered under TRICARE Extra. Users of Standard or Extra can access military medical facilities for free, but unlike Prime enrollees, they receive appointments only when space is available. CBO estimates that there were about 1 million Standard or Extra users in 2012; some of those people relied on civilian health insurance in addition to TRICARE.

Other TRICARE programs are available to subgroups of military beneficiaries, such as those living overseas or in remote locations. One program of note is TRICARE for Life, a wraparound program for military retirees who are eligible for Medicare; it covers the remaining cost of care after Medicare has paid its share. The TFL program is similar to Standard and Extra, but users do not pay TRICARE deductibles or fees. The details of TFL are discussed later in this report.

CBO estimates that the average cost to DoD of providing health care to a Prime enrollee in 2010 (the most recent

---

3. At the time of this writing, 2012 was the most recent year for which DoD had supplied a final tally of the amount of funding provided for the DHP. DoD supplied CBO with preliminary data for 2013, but those data were still subject to change. Overall, funding for 2013 was probably about $5 billion lower than it was in 2012. TRICARE for Life accrual payments equaled $8.3 billion in 2013, versus $10.8 billion in 2012, largely because of more moderate projections of the escalation in future medical costs. In addition, the DHP budget in 2013 was reduced by about $2.3 billion as part of the sequestration of budgetary resources that took place on March 1, 2013, in accordance with the Budget Control Act of 2011.

year for which the data were available) was about $4,800 (in 2014 dollars). For a Standard or Extra user (not including Medicare-eligible users), the average estimated cost was about $3,900.

Historical Funding Trends and Projections of Future Costs

In 1990, military health care accounted for about 4 percent of DoD's base budget—that is, funding for the department's routine activities, excluding funding for overseas contingency operations (OCO), such as the recent operations in Iraq and Afghanistan (see Summary Figure 1 on page 2). DoD created the three plans—Prime, Standard, and Extra—that initially constituted TRICARE in 1993, in anticipation of requirements that would be enacted in the Department of Defense Appropriations Act for Fiscal Year 1994.

Between 1994 and 2000, funding for military health care constituted about 6 percent of DoD's total budget, but that funding has grown rapidly since then, increasing by 130 percent over the past 12 years (from 2000 to 2012), after excluding the effects of overall inflation in the U.S. economy (see Figure 1-2).[4] (Excluding the effects of inflation, that funding had grown by only 14 percent over the previous 10 years, from 1990 to 2000.) As a result, even as overall funding for defense increased sharply, health care funding as a share of those resources rose to almost 10 percent in 2012. By 2028, that share would grow to 11 percent of the cost of implementing DoD's current plans, CBO estimates.

Over the next eight years, DoD's budget, like most other appropriations, will be limited by caps established under the Budget Control Act of 2011 (as modified by the American Taxpayer Relief Act of 2012 and the Bipartisan Budget Act of 2013). In that fiscal climate, growing costs for military health care could constrain DoD's efforts in other areas such as force size, readiness, and weapons modernization.

In its analysis of historical funding trends, CBO used data from DoD's Future Years Defense Program (FYDP) for 2014 through 2018, which the department issued in April 2013. (The FYDP is a historical record of defense forces and spending as well as DoD's plans over the next

five years.)[5] CBO analyzed the seven functional categories in the FYDP that relate to military health care in terms of their size and the extent of their growth since 2000. Three of those categories—purchased care (that is, health care services provided by the private sector through TRICARE contractors), in-house care (provided at military facilities), and accrual payments to finance TRICARE for Life—have accounted for more than 80 percent of the funding for military health care since 2002.

Purchased Health Care, In-House Care, and Accrual Payments

Purchased care cost $15.4 billion in 2012, consuming the largest share of DoD's health care funding (see Figure 1-2). Spending on purchased care more than doubled in the past 12 years, after adjusting for inflation. Because the number of health care providers in the military and the capacity of military treatment facilities have remained essentially fixed over that period, increases in the demand for health care have led to a growing use of, and increased costs for, purchased care.

In-house care provided at military facilities accounted for the next largest share of health care funding, and funding for such care grew by 58 percent above economywide inflation between 2000 and 2012, reaching $15.0 billion in 2012. In that year, about 45 percent of those funds paid for the salaries of military physicians, nurses, and other uniformed providers and administrators. That compensation grew by one-third over the period, implying that other costs associated with in-house care (such as pharmaceuticals and medical supplies) grew by 75 percent.

The annual contributions DoD is required to make to satisfy TFL accrual charges, which are funded from the individual services' military personnel appropriations, grew from about $10 billion to $12 billion (in 2012 dollars) between 2002 and 2007; they have since fallen to about $11 billion in 2012 and $8 billion in 2013.

---

4. To adjust for inflation, CBO used the gross domestic product deflator—the ratio of the value of aggregate domestic output at current prices to its value at base-year prices.

5. The functional categories used in the FYDP offer more detail about how resources are used than do the appropriation titles (military personnel, O&M, and so on) used for the federal budget. Those categories distribute funding among different types of care (for instance, in-house or purchased care) as well as among administrative and ancillary functions. That distribution provides greater insight into the components of DoD's health care funding than do the budget categories shown in Figure 1-1.

Figure 1-2.

Funding for Defense Health Care From DoD's O&M and Military Personnel Appropriations, by Function, 1990 to 2018

(Billions of 2014 dollars)

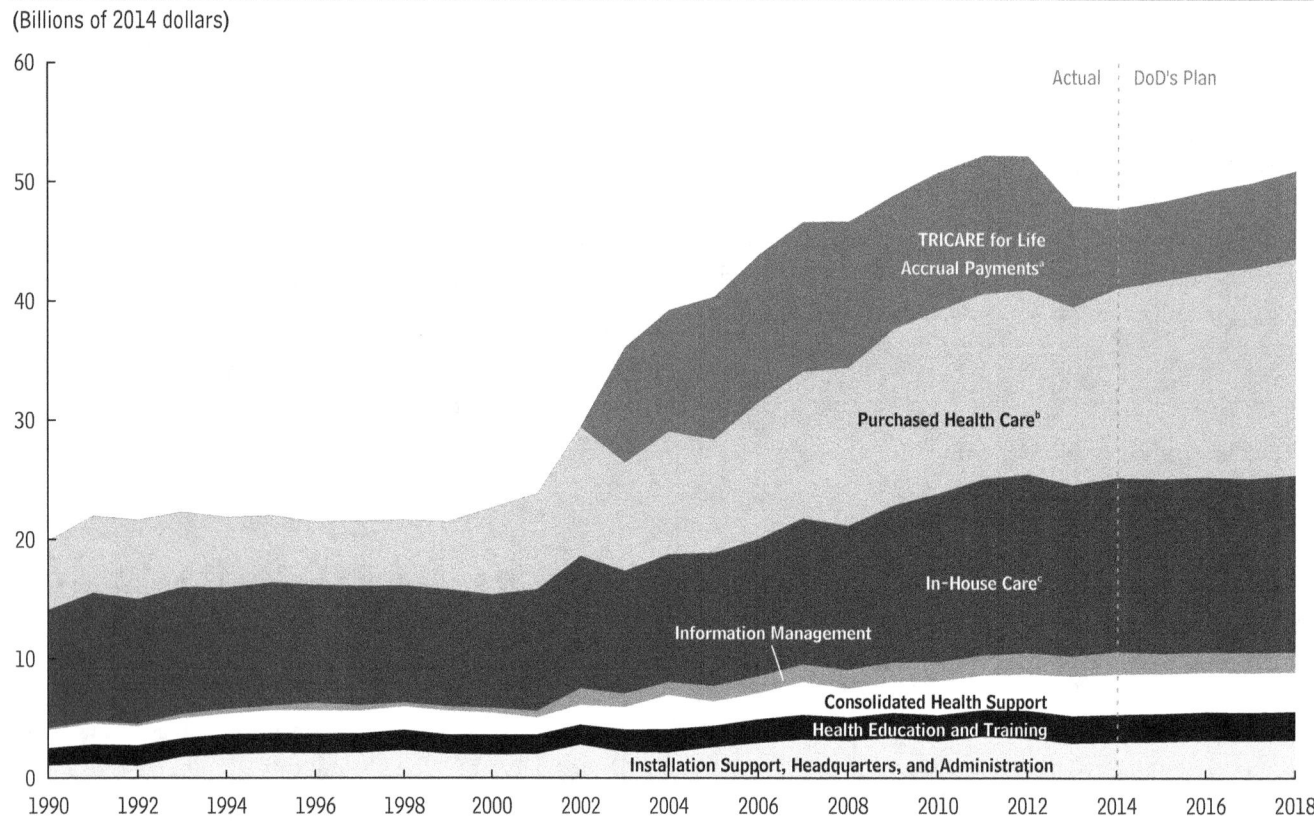

Source: Congressional Budget Office.

Notes: The projection period reflects DoD's plans for the five-year period from 2014 through 2018, as outlined in the 2014 FYDP. Data for 2013 are preliminary.

Supplemental and emergency funding for overseas contingency operations is included for 2013 and preceding years but not for later years. That funding averaged about $1 billion per year from 2002 through 2006 and less than $3 billion per year from 2007 through 2013.

DoD = Department of Defense; O&M = operation and maintenance; FYDP = Future Years Defense Program.

a.   TRICARE for Life accrual payments are made on behalf of all military personnel, not just those who are medical personnel.

b.   Contracted health care provided by the private sector.

c.   Direct health care provided at military facilities.

Other Costs

The remaining 20 percent of funding for military health care finances a variety of activities, including the following:

■ Information management;

■ Consolidated health support, which includes medical laboratories, regional management offices (which oversee the TRICARE regional contractors), public health activities (for example, tobacco-cessation campaigns), care for working animals, and aeromedical evacuations;

■ Health education and training programs, which provide medical education and training both through DoD-operated activities and through scholarships; and

■ Installation support—that is, maintaining, sustaining, restoring, and modernizing the clinics, hospitals, and associated buildings on military installations—plus headquarters and administrative functions.

All told, funding for those activities rose by 78 percent (excluding the effects of inflation) from 2000 to 2012 and totaled $10 billion in 2012.

Causes of Past Increases in Health Care Costs

Because the bulk of military health care funding is for purchased care, in-house care, and accrual payments, CBO analyzed causes of those past increases to identify approaches to reduce future spending. Most researchers and policymakers suggest three reasons that the growth in military health care costs has far outpaced growth in the broader U.S. economy:

- *New and expanded TRICARE benefits.* A decade of legislative changes has added new groups of beneficiaries and expanded access for existing beneficiaries.

- *Increased utilization fostered by financial incentives to use TRICARE.* Beneficiaries' cost-sharing burden has been declining, so TRICARE has become increasingly attractive when compared with other options for health care coverage.

- *Medical costs of recent wars.* More than 50,000 U.S. military personnel have been wounded during the operations in Iraq and Afghanistan, and many will bear the effects of those injuries for years. Because the number of wounded service members is smaller than the number of new beneficiaries using TRICARE, and because most of those who served in Iraq and Afghanistan will leave (or have already left) active service, those operations have increased medical costs in the base budget for the DHP by less than the factors described in the preceding two paragraphs. Providing care to wounded veterans may add to the costs of the Veterans Health Administration, but those costs are not included in this analysis of DoD's health care system.

New and Expanded TRICARE Benefits

Since 2000, lawmakers have authorized and DoD has implemented a number of changes to the TRICARE program that have expanded the pool of eligible beneficiaries. Between 2000 and 2012, the number of eligible beneficiaries grew by an average of about 1 percent per year, rising from 8.2 million to 9.1 million (see Figure 1-3).[6] Much of that increase occurred between 2001 and 2003,

in part because of the start of the TRICARE for Life program. That program also accounts for some of the growth beyond 2003.

Another reason for the increase between 2001 and 2003 was the rise in mobilizations and deployments of National Guard and Reserve personnel during the first few years after September 11, 2001. At the time, those reservists became eligible for TRICARE only after they had served on active duty for more than 30 days, and their eligibility ended when they were demobilized. Although those deployments slowed in the middle of the decade, the number of eligible beneficiaries did not decline proportionally because another new benefit created by lawmakers—TRICARE Reserve Select— allowed them to remain. The increase in the number of Army and Marine Corps personnel was largely offset by reductions in the Navy and the Air Force, so that the number of active-duty members and their families remained relatively constant over the period.

TRICARE for Life. Military personnel who serve on active duty for 20 years or more, or who become medically disabled while serving, are eligible to retire. However, because most service members join the military between the ages of 18 and 25, few are old enough to qualify for Medicare immediately upon retirement; at that point, military retirees under the age of 65 can continue to participate in TRICARE or obtain health care from other sources.

TRICARE for Life is designed as a wraparound program for military retirees who are eligible for Medicare.[7] TFL requires beneficiaries to enroll in Medicare Part B, which

---

6. Because this study focuses on DoD, data for eligible members of the Coast Guard and for the commissioned corps of the Public Health Service and the National Oceanic and Atmospheric Administration (and their families) are excluded from the totals used in this chapter.

7. Between 1966, when Medicare began to provide benefits, and 2002, when TRICARE for Life went into effect, military retirees who became eligible for Medicare could not use TRICARE (or its predecessor program); 86 percent of them purchased supplemental insurance to cover the costs that Medicare would not. See Department of Defense, *Evaluation of the TRICARE Program—Access, Cost and Quality: Fiscal Year 2013 Report to Congress* (February 2013), p. 87, http://go.usa.gov/jX9H. Medicare-eligible beneficiaries were still able to seek free medical care from military providers, but only if space was available after other patients were seen.

Figure 1-3.

Number of DoD Beneficiaries Eligible for TRICARE, 2000 to 2012

(Millions of people)

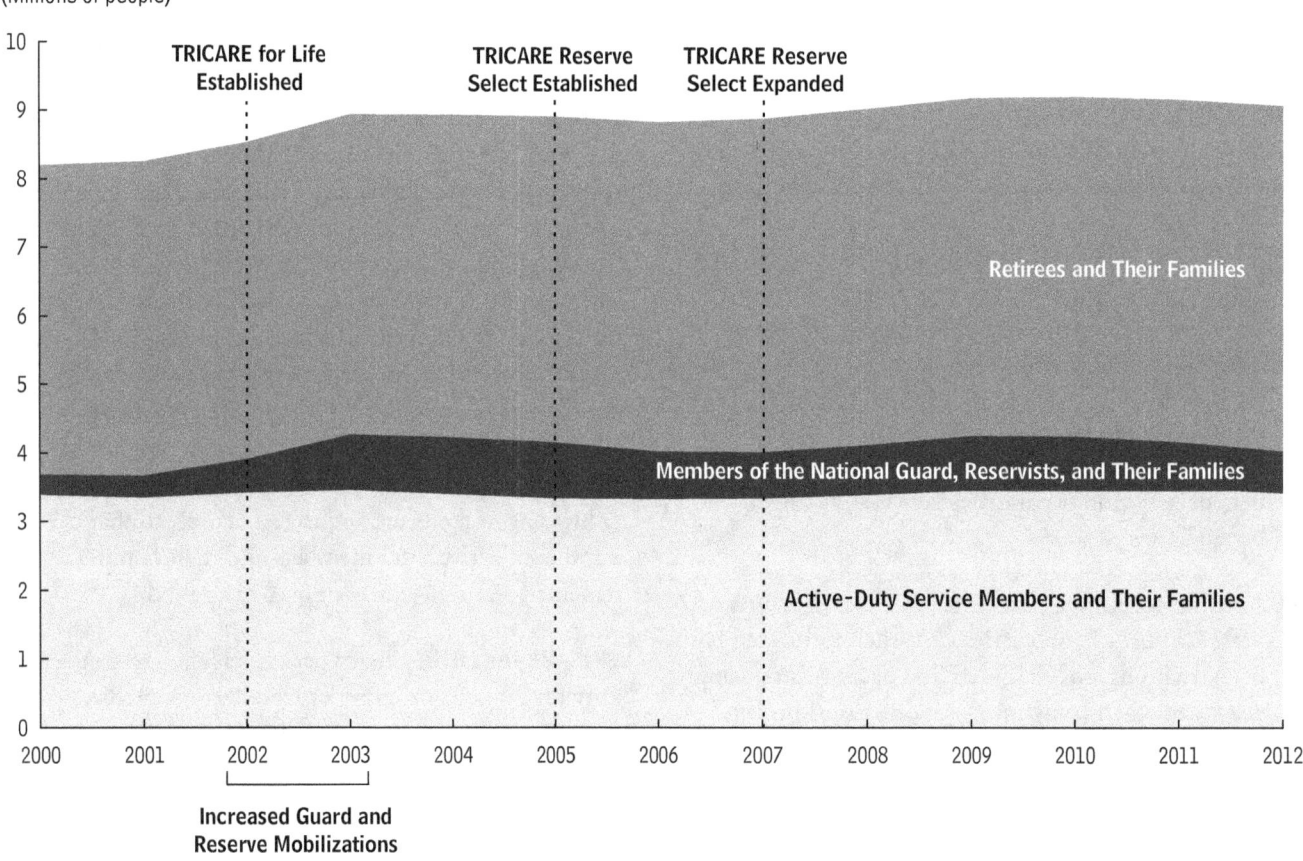

Source: Congressional Budget Office.

Notes: Excludes eligible members of the Coast Guard and the commissioned corps of the Public Health Service and of the National Oceanic and Atmospheric Administration (and their families).

DoD = Department of Defense.

charges annual premiums based on income, but TFL charges no annual premium or enrollment fee for the wraparound benefit itself. For services that are covered by both Medicare and TRICARE, Medicare pays first, and TFL pays the remaining balance. For services not covered by Medicare, TFL is the first payer. Thus, TFL largely eliminates the out-of-pocket costs for retirees and their families. DoD reports that about 1.6 million people enrolled in TFL in 2012.[8]

TRICARE for Life is financed differently from other defense health programs. DoD pays what actuaries esti-

mate to be the amount necessary to fund future health care benefits for members currently serving in the military. In 2013, those accrual payments to the MERHCF amounted to $8.3 billion. That same year, the outlays from the fund to reimburse TRICARE contract providers and military treatment facilities for care delivered to current Medicare-eligible retirees totaled $8.2 billion. Those two sums usually differ in any given year because the former is an estimate of future costs for current service members, whereas the latter measures current costs for people who have already retired from the military.

The anticipated future cost of TFL is substantial, in part, because its beneficiaries generally will be at least age 65 and are expected to use far more health care services than active-duty members or working-age retirees (who are not

---

8.   Department of Defense, *Evaluation of the TRICARE Program— Access, Cost and Quality: Fiscal Year 2013 Report to Congress* (February 2013), p. 16, http://go.usa.gov/jX9H.

Figure 1-4.

Per Capita Use of TRICARE by Retirees and Their Families Relative to Use by Active-Duty Service Members and Their Families, 2010

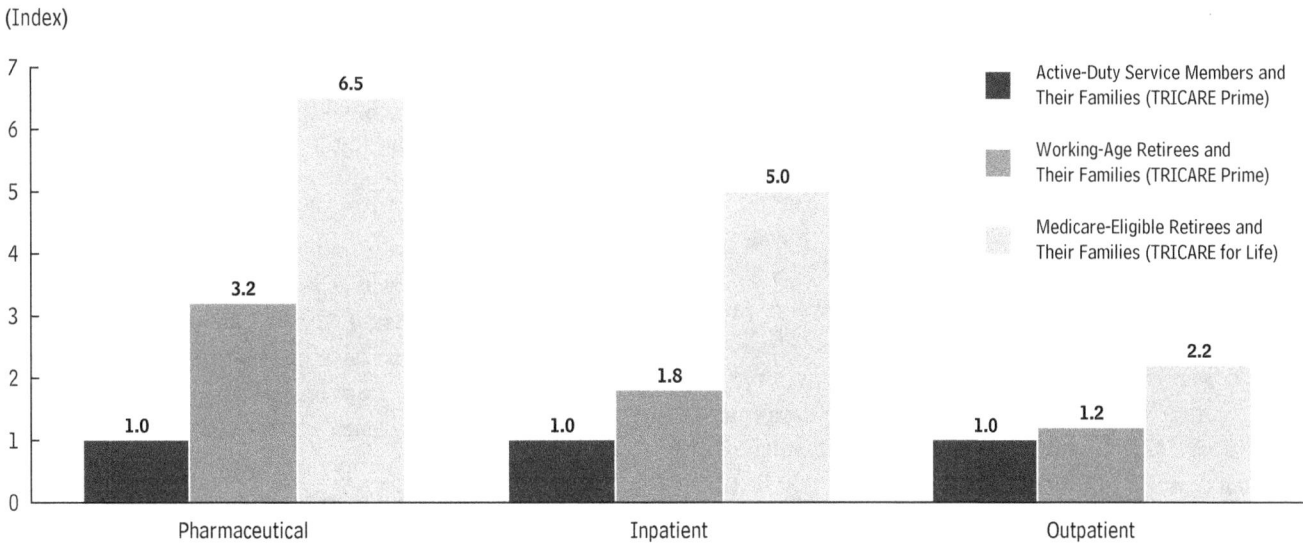

Source: Congressional Budget Office.

Notes: Use of pharmaceutical, inpatient, and outpatient services by active-duty service members and their families has been normalized to 1 to serve as a benchmark against which to compare use by working-age and Medicare-eligible retirees and their families.

Pharmaceutical use is measured as the number of 30-day equivalent prescriptions per member per year.

Inpatient utilization (that is, treatment requiring admittance to a hospital or other acute care facility) is measured as the relative weighted products (RWPs) per 1,000 people. An RWP ranks the resources used to provide acute care on a common scale by weighting the average cost per inpatient stay by the complexity of the patient's condition. RWPs more accurately reflect differences across beneficiary groups than discharges per capita because they adjust for the intensity of care required.

Outpatient usage (that is, visits for treatments or procedures not requiring hospitalization) is measured by relative value units (RVUs) per person per year. RVUs rank the resources used to provide a service on a common scale. An outpatient visit for primary care has an average RVU value of about 1.5.

eligible for Medicare) and their respective families. For instance, in 2010, working-age retirees and their families obtained more than three times as many 30-day prescriptions per user as active-duty members and their families; but TFL users obtained more than six times as many (see Figure 1-4). Inpatient usage (that is, treatment requiring admittance to a hospital or other acute care facility) among Medicare-eligible retirees was almost three times greater than that of working-age retirees and their families and five times greater than usage by active-duty members and their families.[9] Outpatient usage (that is, visits for treatments or procedures not requiring hospitalization) varied the least among the three groups; working-age retirees consumed about 25 percent more outpatient services than active-duty members and their families, and TFL users consumed about twice the amount.[10] That higher usage in TFL for all categories of

care is not surprising because TFL users are older and prone to more health concerns than other beneficiaries

9. Mail-order prescriptions provide a 90-day supply; most other prescriptions are for a 30-day supply. The mail-order data have been adjusted to derive the number of "30-day-equivalent" prescriptions. Inpatient usage is measured as relative weighted products (RWPs) per 1,000 people. RWPs more accurately reflect differences across beneficiary groups than discharges per capita because they adjust for the intensity of care required. A complex hospitalization lasting several days will have a larger RWP than a shorter hospital stay.

10. Outpatient usage is measured by the number of relative value units (RVUs) per person per year. RVUs measure the relative resources consumed by a single visit as compared with the average of all visits, so that a very complicated procedure has a higher RVU value than a simple visit. An outpatient visit for primary care takes an average RVU value of about 1.5.

and because their out-of-pocket expenses are generally smaller.

TRICARE Reserve Select. Over the past seven years, lawmakers have also expanded TRICARE coverage for members of the National Guard and Reserve by authorizing the TRICARE Reserve Select (TRS) program. Before 2005, reservists or guardsmen (and their dependents) were eligible for TRICARE only if they served on active duty for more than 30 days. They remained eligible only as long as they remained on active duty. Since 2005, under the TRS program, eligible members of the National Guard and Reserve have been allowed to purchase TRICARE Standard and Extra coverage. To be eligible, members had to have served on active duty (been "activated") for at least 90 consecutive days since September 11, 2001, in support of overseas combat operations like those in Iraq and Afghanistan. In 2007, this premium-based program was expanded to include almost all reservists and guard members.[11] The premium is designed to cover 28 percent of the estimated cost of the program. Although the TRS program is still small, its use has increased almost fivefold—from 35,000 enrollees (including dependents) at the end of 2007 to more than 240,000 enrollees at the end of 2011.[12] One study suggests that TRS enrollment could increase substantially after 2014 because the premium compares favorably with the expected premiums (net of subsidies) for plans in the health insurance exchanges established under the Affordable Care Act.[13] In addition, that study noted that TRS premiums are only slightly higher than the penalty for not having insurance. Thus, the number of TRS enrollees may continue to increase in the future.

---

11. Any member of the Selected Reserve (that is, a member of the Reserve who drills regularly, not just one who has served in overseas combat operations) can join the TRS program as long as he or she is not eligible for the Federal Employees Health Benefits program.

12. Department of Defense, *Evaluation of the TRICARE Program— Access, Cost and Quality: Fiscal Year 2013 Report to Congress* (February 2013), p. 44, http://go.usa.gov/jX9H.

13. See Susan D. Hosek, *Healthcare Coverage and Disability Evaluation for Reserve Component Personnel: Research for the 11th Quadrennial Review of Military Compensation* (RAND Corporation, 2012), www.rand.org/pubs/monographs/MG1157. The Affordable Care Act comprises the Patient Protection and Affordable Care Act and the amendments made to that law by the health care provisions of the Health Care and Education Reconciliation Act of 2010.

Increased Utilization Fostered by Financial Incentives to Use TRICARE

The share of health care costs paid by TRICARE users is smaller than that paid by most civilian consumers using private health insurance. That disparity has been growing because, since the mid-1990s, most of TRICARE's fees have decreased, or increased only slightly; by contrast, premiums and cost sharing for civilian health plans have tended to increase at least as rapidly as per capita health care costs nationwide. TRICARE's comparatively low out-of-pocket costs have had two effects: First, the number of users has increased as people have switched from more expensive plans to TRICARE; and second, TRICARE participants have increased the volume of health services they consume. DoD's per-beneficiary costs for the military health system—not including TFL accrual charges, which apply to future beneficiaries— have increased by more than 60 percent in real (inflation-adjusted) terms since 2000, rising from $2,800 in 2000 to $4,500 in 2012, measured in 2014 dollars (see Figure 1-5).[14]

Prices Paid by TRICARE Users. Enrollment fees, co-payments, and deductibles for TRICARE users are significantly lower than the corresponding fees for most civilian plans. (See the appendix for the current cost-sharing schedules.) For example, military retirees can purchase family coverage in Prime for significantly less than they could in a typical HMO offered in the civilian sector (see Table 1-1). DoD has estimated that, in 2012, a typical military retiree could purchase Prime coverage for $520 per year and would, on average, pay another $445 in copayments and other fees, for a total annual cost of $965. By contrast, DoD estimated that a civilian in the general U.S. population who enrolled in a family HMO plan offered by an employer would typically pay $5,080 in premiums (not including any share paid by the employer); with deductibles and copayments averaging $1,000, that family would pay a total of $6,080 over the course of a year. Thus, a family enrolled in TRICARE

---

14. Because TRICARE Standard and Extra do not require enrollment, DoD could not provide data on the number of people using those plans between 2000 and 2012. Figure 1-5 depicts the cost per eligible beneficiary, but because about 20 percent of people who are eligible for TRICARE do not use the benefit, the actual per-user cost of providing health care differs from the values shown.

Figure 1-5.

Funding for Defense Health Care per Eligible TRICARE Beneficiary

(2014 dollars)

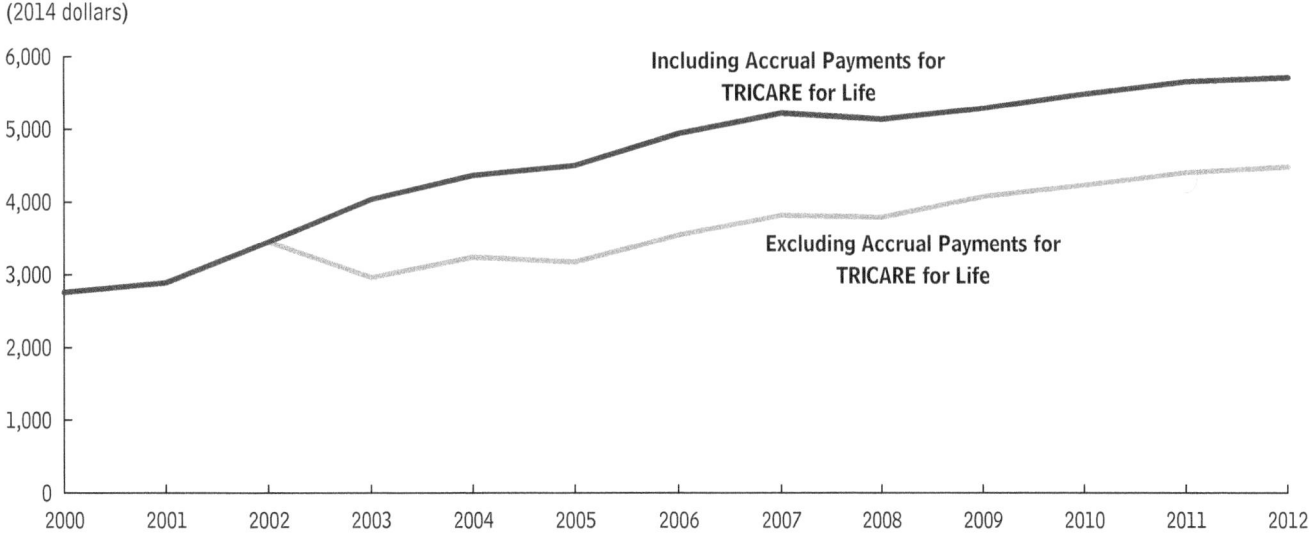

Source: Congressional Budget Office.

Notes: This figure reflects the Department of Defense's spending for health care from its appropriations for operation and maintenance and military personnel.

Not all people who are eligible to use TRICARE do so; consequently, this measure is lower than the Department of Defense's spending per user.

Data on the number of users (as distinct from eligible beneficiaries) are not available for the entire 2000–2012 period.

Prime would pay about one-sixth of what a similar family would pay for coverage in a civilian HMO.[15] A family who used Standard or Extra, which require no enrollment fees, would pay about one-fifth of what a similar family would pay for coverage in a civilian preferred provider organization.

Enrollment fees for TRICARE did not change between 1995 and 2010 and have increased only slightly since then. In contrast, for most civilian plans, the employee's share of employment-based health insurance premiums

---

15. Department of Defense, *Evaluation of the TRICARE Program—Access, Cost and Quality: Fiscal Year 2013 Report to Congress* (February 2013), pp. 83 and 85, http://go.usa.gov/jX9H. An independent source shows amounts similar to those estimated by DoD and reported here; see Kaiser Family Foundation and Health Research and Educational Trust, *Employer Health Benefits Survey: 2013 Summary of Findings* (September 2013), http://tinyurl.com/oldtycg. According to that survey, the average employee's share of the premium for a family HMO plan and a family preferred provider organization plan was $5,125 and $4,590, respectively, in 2013 (p. 2). DoD adjusted the civilian data to match the age distribution and the average family size of the TRICARE population, so its estimates differed from the results of the Kaiser Survey.

and the premiums of privately purchased insurance have grown annually since 2000. Copayments and other out-of-pocket expenses rose for civilians as well. Because TRICARE's fees have remained largely fixed, with only modest increases starting in 2010, the attractiveness of TRICARE as an alternative to private and other government plans has grown.

In addition, several policy changes over the past decade have made TRICARE even more financially appealing. In 2000, DoD reduced the catastrophic cap—the maximum out-of-pocket liability per family for copayments, cost sharing, and deductibles over the course of a fiscal year—under TRICARE Standard from $7,500 to $3,000 for military retirees and their families. In 2001, DoD eliminated copayments for outpatient visits to TRICARE Prime providers by the family members of active-duty personnel. Those copayments had been $6 for the families of junior enlisted personnel (pay grades E-4 and below) and $12 for all others.

Rising Number of TRICARE Users. The total number of active-duty members, working-age retirees (that is, those who are not yet eligible for Medicare), and family

Table 1-1.

Average Annual Costs of Family Coverage Incurred by Military Retirees and Their Civilian Counterparts With Employment-Based Insurance, 2012

(Dollars)

Plan	Premium or Enrollment Fee	Deductibles and Copayments	Total Annual Costs per Family
TRICARE Prime	520	445	965
Civilian HMO	5,080	1,000	6,080
TRICARE as a percentage of civilian plan			16
TRICARE Standard or Extra	0	1,035	1,035
Civilian PPO	4,270	1,295	5,565
TRICARE as a percentage of civilian plan			19

Source: Department of Defense, *Evaluation of the TRICARE Program—Access, Cost, and Quality: Fiscal Year 2013 Report to Congress* (February 2013), pp. 83 and 85.

Notes: The Department of Defense adjusted the civilian data to match the age-and-sex distribution and the average family size of the TRICARE population.

HMO = health maintenance organization; PPO = preferred provider organization.

members who were *eligible* for TRICARE rose by 4 percent between 2003 and 2012 (see Table 1-2). The number of users *enrolled* in Prime increased faster—by 8 percent—over the same period. Both the number of active-duty personnel (and their family members) and the percentage who enrolled in Prime have been relatively stable. By contrast, both the number of working-age retirees (and their family members) who are eligible for TRICARE and the percentage who enrolled in Prime rose significantly over that period. Their numbers grew by 400,000 (or 13 percent) between 2003 and 2012, reaching a total of 3.5 million. The proportion who joined Prime grew from 39 percent in 2003 to 46 percent in 2012. The net result of those two trends was that working-age retirees and their family members accounted for effectively all of the 400,000 additional beneficiaries who enrolled in Prime between 2003 and 2012. Most of those people had access to other types of health insurance (such as insurance offered through a current employer or a spouse's employer), but they chose to enroll in TRICARE.

Quantity of Health Care Services Consumed. The degree to which consumers share in the overall cost of health care services tends to affect the quantity of services they buy.[16] DoD estimates that in 2012 the average person enrolled in Prime used 50 percent more outpatient services than the average civilian in an HMO.[17]

Data provided by DoD for the years 2005 through 2010 suggest that per capita use of outpatient and pharmacy services increased by more than 20 percent during that period (see Figure 1-6). The use of inpatient services per person, however, has remained roughly constant.[18] About 70 percent to 80 percent of medical care is delivered by private contractors in the form of purchased care. Most of the growth in outpatient utilization has occurred in purchased care; the in-house system has maintained a relatively constant workload since 2005.

---

16. See Willard Manning and others, "Health Insurance and the Demand for Medical Care: Evidence From a Randomized Experiment," *American Economic Review,* vol. 77, no. 3 (1987), pp. 251–277; Robert H. Brook and others, "Does Free Care Improve Adults' Health? Results from a Randomized Controlled Trial," *New England Journal of Medicine,* vol. 309, no. 23 (1983), pp. 1426–1434; and Katherine Swartz, *Cost-Sharing: Effects on Spending and Outcomes,* Research Synthesis Report No. 20 (Robert Wood Johnson Foundation, December 2010), http://tinyurl.com/oyle4s8.

17. DoD adjusted the civilian data to match the age-and-sex distribution of the TRICARE population. See Department of Defense, *Evaluation of the Tricare Program—Access, Cost and Quality: Fiscal Year 2013 Report to Congress* (February 2013), p. 72, http://go.usa.gov/jX9H.

18. Indexes for inpatient, outpatient, and pharmacy use are measured the same way as in earlier portions of the analysis (see footnotes 9 and 10). But, in this instance, CBO combined the data across all types of beneficiaries and measured the change relative to 2005 for each type of care.

Table 1-2.

Enrollment in TRICARE Prime by Type of Beneficiary, 2003 and 2012

	Total Number of People Eligible to Enroll in TRICARE Prime (Millions)	Number of Eligible Beneficiaries Enrolled in TRICARE Prime (Millions)	Percentage of Eligible Beneficiaries Enrolled in TRICARE Prime
2003			
Active-Duty Service Members	1.8	1.8	100
Families of Active-Duty Service Members	2.4	1.9	79
Working-Age Retirees and Their Families	3.1	1.2	39
Total	**7.3**	**4.9**	**67**
2012			
Active-Duty Service Members	1.7	1.7	100
Families of Active-Duty Service Members	2.4	2.0	83
Working-Age Retirees and Their Families	3.5	1.6	46
Total	**7.6**	**5.3**	**70**

Source: Department of Defense, *Evaluation of the TRICARE Program—Access, Cost, and Quality: Fiscal Year 2013 Report to Congress* (February 2013), p. 16, and *Evaluation of the TRICARE Program, Fiscal Year 2005 Report to Congress* (March 2005), p. 20.

Notes: Data for people who are not eligible to enroll in TRICARE Prime—particularly members of the National Guard, reservists, and Medicare-eligible beneficiaries, and their respective families—are not included in this table.

Data reflect the average number of people in each year to account for beneficiaries who were eligible or enrolled for only a part of a year.

Medical Costs of Recent Wars

Several war-related factors affect the need for military health care. First, more people are deployed to hostile environments, and their overall health must be evaluated and any shortcomings remedied before they can go. Second, more people are injured in combat. In addition to physical injuries, the demand for military health care has increased because of the growing incidence of post-traumatic stress disorder and traumatic brain injury and the need to better assess the mental health of those returning from Iraq and Afghanistan.[19]

The Defense Health Program and the military medical departments—commanded by the Surgeons General of

the Army, Navy, and Air Force—have complementary responsibilities during wars. Health care needed in the midst of combat is provided by the military departments. Thus, the care provided in Iraq and Afghanistan at battle-aid stations or on Navy hospital ships cannot explain increasing costs for the DHP. However, established military hospitals overseas—for example, the military hospital in Landstuhl, Germany, where most serious casualties from Iraq and Afghanistan are treated before being transported back to the United States—are funded as part of the DHP, as are U.S. facilities, such as the Walter Reed National Military Medical Center, where many wounded service members receive rehabilitative care.

Funds related to combat and casualty care can be provided in three ways:

■ Through appropriations that are tied to specific contingencies (which may include humanitarian operations as well as military action);

---

19. Much of the cost of caring for post-traumatic stress disorder and traumatic brain injury falls to the Veterans Health Administration, and not DoD. See Congressional Budget Office, *The Veterans Health Administration's Treatment of PTSD and Traumatic Brain Injury Among Recent Combat Veterans* (February 2012), www.cbo.gov/publication/42969.

Figure 1-6.

Per Capita Use of TRICARE by All Beneficiaries

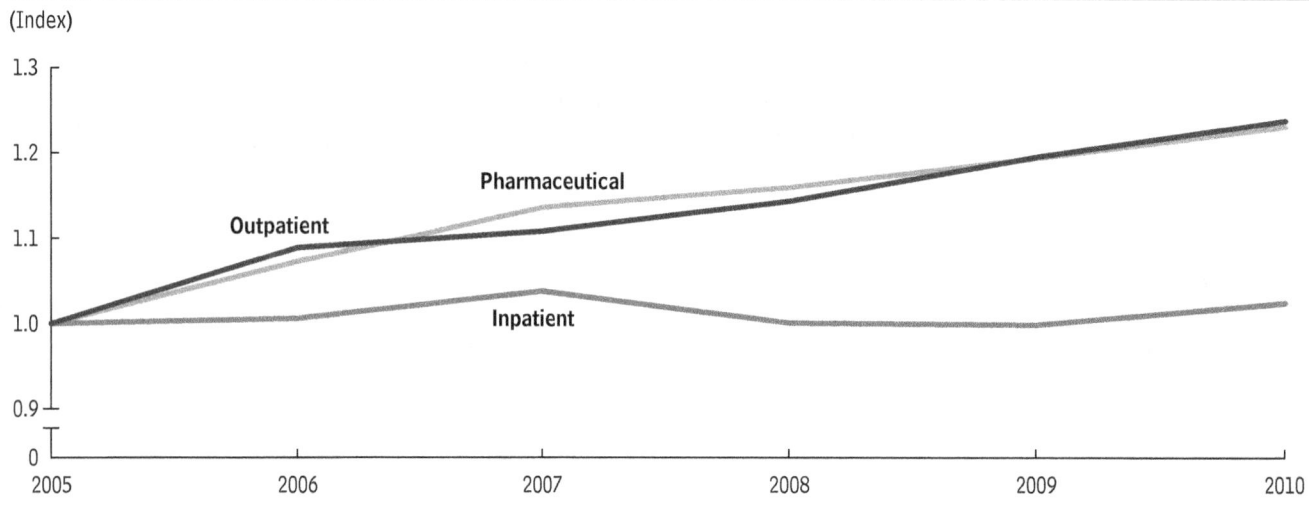

Source: Congressional Budget Office.

Notes: Data are measured relative to levels of use in 2005 to allow depiction on a single graph.

Eligible beneficiaries include active-duty service members, working-age retirees, Medicare-eligible retirees, and their respective families.

Pharmaceutical use is measured as the number of 30-day equivalent prescriptions per member per year.

Inpatient utilization (that is, treatment requiring admittance to a hospital or other acute care facility) is measured as the relative weighted products (RWPs) per 1,000 people. An RWP ranks the resources used to provide acute care on a common scale by weighting the average cost per inpatient stay by the complexity of the patient's condition. RWPs more accurately reflect differences across beneficiary groups than discharges per capita because they adjust for the intensity of care required.

Outpatient usage (that is, visits for treatments or procedures not requiring hospitalization) is measured by relative value units (RVUs) per person per year. RVUs rank the resources used to provide a service on a common scale. An outpatient visit for primary care takes an average RVU value of about 1.5.

■ Through war-related appropriations in the annual base budget; or

■ Through the regular DHP appropriation.

Funding for contingencies and other war-related activities represents a relatively small portion of the DHP's overall budget. Moreover, the care of all active-duty personnel represents a small part of overall health care provided to all beneficiaries. For those two reasons, CBO finds that wartime requirements explain relatively little of the growth in the DHP's funding since 2000.

Funding From Specific Contingency-Related Appropriations. Most of the funding for overseas contingency operations, particularly for the wars in Afghanistan and Iraq, has come from emergency and supplemental appropriations outside of DoD's base-budget request.[20] (The DHP also received supplemental funding for humanitarian missions, such as those following the earthquake in Haiti in 2010, but those funds were not

included in CBO's analysis.) Between 2002 and 2009, OCO funding represented between 4 percent and 11 percent of total annual O&M funding for the DHP. That percentage was about 4 percent from 2010 through 2012, as U.S. forces withdrew from Iraq.[21] At $1.3 billion in 2012, in 2014 dollars, OCO funding for the DHP accounted for only a small fraction of the growth in that program since 2000.

20. Starting in 2002, funds for wartime operations were requested by the President and appropriated by the Congress in legislation that was supplemental to legislation that provided funding for regular defense operations (or base budgets). Since February 2010, the President's budget request has included—but separately identified—the OCO funds for fiscal years 2011 through 2014. The Congress, in turn, has thus far provided OCO funding and base-budget funding in the same bills for each of those years through 2013.

21. These numbers do not include OCO funds appropriated to pay for the TFL accrual payments for activated guard members and reservists.

Figure 1-7.

Contingency-Related Funding for the Defense Health Program

(Billions of 2014 dollars)

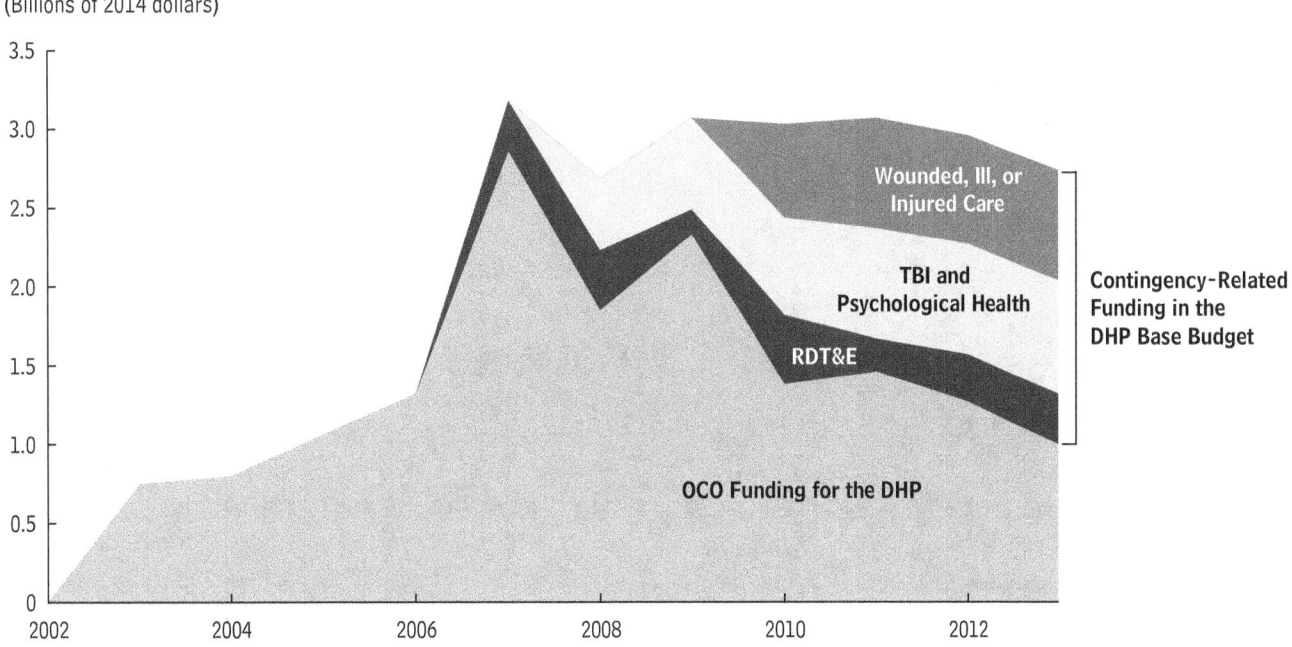

Source: Congressional Budget Office based on data from the Department of Defense.

Notes: The base budget for the DHP includes funding for DoD's routine health-related activities, excluding funding for operations in Iraq and Afghanistan. The DHP has received additional appropriations to support health care costs associated with overseas contingency operations, including operations in Iraq and Afghanistan.

Care for the wounded, ill, or injured was included in OCO funding from 2007 to 2009 and identified separately in regular budget requests beginning in 2010.

Funding for the treatment of traumatic brain injuries and psychological health reported by DoD in 2008 also includes funding for those programs in 2006 and 2007.

These data do not include the costs of care provided in combat areas by the military departments directly because those costs are not part of the DHP.

Data for 2013 are preliminary.

TBI = traumatic brain injury; DHP = Defense Health Program; RDT&E = research, development, test, and evaluation; OCO = overseas contingency operations; DoD = Department of Defense.

War-Related Funding in the Base Budget. In addition to OCO funds received to support overseas contingencies, DoD has identified some funds (amounting to less than $2 billion annually since 2007 in 2014 dollars) in the DHP's base budget that are related to the decade of sustained conflict (see Figure 1-7).[22] Funding for the care of wounded, ill, and injured personnel ($690 million in 2012) is designed to support case management, the disability evaluation system, data sharing with the Department of Veterans Affairs, and similar programs.

---

22. Department of Defense, *Evaluation of the TRICARE Program—Access, Cost and Quality: Fiscal Year 2013 Report to Congress* (February 2013), p.18, http://go.usa.gov/jX9H.

Specific initiatives to treat traumatic brain injuries and mental health have been funded separately, amounting to $700 million in 2012. DoD also received some war-related funding (about $300 million in 2012) for research and development. War-related funding may continue into future years, but that funding represents a relatively small part of the defense health care budget and is not likely to contribute to future growth.

Funding the Care of Active-Duty Personnel in the Regular DHP Appropriation. The people who may potentially engage in combat—those serving on active duty—represent a relatively small portion of all TRICARE beneficiaries, and they tend to use the system less than other groups. Also, their numbers have remained relatively constant despite a decade of war.[23] About 9.7 million people were eligible to use TRICARE in 2012. Of those, about 1.7 million were active-duty service members, including some activated members of the National Guard and Reserve. During most of the period since 2002, fewer than 300,000 military personnel were deployed in support of the conflicts in Iraq and Afghanistan at any point in time. As of December 2012, about 140,000 personnel were deployed for those overseas contingency operations.[24] Through December 2013, more than 58,500 military personnel had been wounded in the operations in Iraq and Afghanistan.

Besides being a small portion of all TRICARE beneficiaries, active-duty personnel also use fewer services than other groups. CBO estimates that, in 2010, active-duty members' inpatient stays occurred at a rate of about one-quarter less than that for their family members and about half the rate for working-age retirees and their families.[25] The top two inpatient diagnoses in terms of volume and cost (in military and private-sector hospitals combined) were related to childbirth, which involves family members far more often than it does active-duty members themselves.[26]

In 2010, the average active-duty member filled about two-thirds the number of prescriptions that an average family member did. The use (per person) of outpatient services by active-duty personnel, however, was about 20 percent higher than among their family members. That basic relationship—active-duty personnel using fewer inpatient facilities and prescriptions but more outpatient services than their family members—has existed since 2003. DoD reports, however, that the number of outpatient visits by active-duty personnel was about equal to the usage by active-duty families between 2000 and 2002, the period just before the overseas contingency operations began.[27] Casualty care, health assessments both before and after deployment, and other care associated with wartime may account for some of the increased use of outpatient services by active-duty personnel since 2003, but the data provided by DoD do not allow CBO to quantify the effect.

Projections for 2014 Through 2028

In CBO's projection of DoD's plans, which is based on the department's 2014 Future Years Defense Program, the department's health care costs rise from $49 billion in 2014 to $70 billion in 2028 (in 2014 dollars), an increase of about 40 percent, excluding the effects of inflation; as a share of DoD's total resources, health care costs are projected to increase from 9 percent to 11 percent.[28] That increase is expected to result mostly from rising per capita costs, rather than from changes in the number of TRICARE users. Using DoD's projections of its eligible beneficiary population, CBO estimates that the number of TRICARE users will remain approximately constant, even declining a bit by 2028 as the large cohort of retirees associated with the substantial force levels maintained during the Cold War gradually gets smaller and is replaced by the smaller cohort of retirees that served on active duty after 1995. Implicit in this estimate is the assumption that neither lawmakers nor DoD will institute new benefits that will expand the eligible TRICARE population or the costs of the program.

Because future funding for overseas contingency operations will depend on how conditions evolve in Afghanistan and on whether new contingencies or humanitarian emergencies arise elsewhere, CBO did not include costs of additional overseas operations (beyond the spending of actual appropriations through 2013) in its estimates.

23. Although the Army and the Marine Corps experienced increases in the number of personnel over the past decade, reductions in the number of Navy and Air Force personnel offset those increases, so the total number of active-duty personnel has remained relatively steady since 2000.

24. Department of Defense, Defense Manpower Data Center, "Active Duty Military Personnel by Service by Region/Country," *Military Personnel Statistics* (accessed December 23, 2013), www.dmdc.osd.mil/appj/dwp/reports.do?category=reports &subCat=milActDutReg.

25. Those figures include only those beneficiaries enrolled in Prime. Inpatient utilization is measured as RWPs per 1,000 people per year, as it was in the previous section.

26. Department of Defense, *Evaluation of the TRICARE Program— Access, Cost and Quality: Fiscal Year 2013 Report to Congress* (February 2013), p. 71, http://go.usa.gov/jX9H.

27. Department of Defense, *Evaluation of the TRICARE Program: Fiscal Year 2003 Report to Congress* (October 2003), p. 41, http://go.usa.gov/j5hP.

28. Congressional Budget Office, *Long-Term Implications of the Fiscal Year 2014 Future Years Defense Program* (November 2013), p. 24, www.cbo.gov/publication/44683.

Per capita costs for TRICARE, however, are projected to increase significantly because out-of-pocket costs borne by TRICARE users will continue to increase more slowly than health care costs nationwide, a trend that will keep usage rates for health care higher for TRICARE users than for comparable civilians. For the 2014–2018 period, CBO projects that real per capita spending for TRICARE would grow by an average of 4.8 percent per year if the program remains unchanged. CBO projects that pay and benefits for military personnel who work in the military health system will increase at the same rate as for other military personnel. CBO projected the costs of direct care and administration, purchased care and contracts, and pharmaceuticals between 2014 and 2018 starting from DoD's 2014 FYDP but with two upward adjustments. First, CBO added an annual increase of 1 percent to the costs of direct care because DoD's projection that such costs will be unchanged in real terms over the FYDP period is not consistent with historical experience. Also, to be consistent with current law, CBO excluded the Administration's estimates of savings in purchased care and pharmacy costs that would result from initiatives

related to beneficiary cost sharing that DoD proposed but that the Congress did not adopt in the National Defense Authorization Act for Fiscal Year 2014.

CBO estimated that, after 2018, the per capita costs of military health care would grow at the same rates that the agency projects for health care nationwide, apart from Medicare (because that program differs in important ways from the rest of the nation's health care system).[29] On that basis, the entire 2014–2028 period, annual real growth rates per user in the military health system would average 1.9 percent for direct care and administration, 3.3 percent for purchased care and contracts, and 3.0 percent for pharmaceuticals.

---

29. Congressional Budget Office, *The 2013 Long-Term Budget Outlook* (September 2013), p. 53, www.cbo.gov/publication/44521. CBO's estimates using this approach are very similar to those that would result from applying DoD-specific excess growth factors to the National Health Expenditure projections developed by the Centers for Medicare & Medicaid Services: *National Health Expenditure Projections, 2011–2021*, http://go.usa.gov/WD9V.

Alternatives for Reducing DoD's Health Care Spending

Many policymakers—both inside and outside of the Department of Defense—have expressed concern that rising health care costs will reduce the resources available to fund other activities related to national defense. Those who have studied the military health care system as well as broader issues associated with federal spending for health care have identified several approaches that could reduce the system's spending. The Congressional Budget Office examined three of those approaches:

■ *Improve patients' health by better managing chronic diseases.* Disease management programs could potentially reduce spending by providing less-expensive preventive or routine care as a means of reducing more-costly acute care.

■ *Administer the military health care system more effectively.* DoD could close its in-house medical school and rely more on scholarships to recruit prospective medical professionals while training them at civilian universities. It could also increase its efforts to reduce fraud by expanding its auditing services.

■ *Increase cost sharing for retirees who use TRICARE.* DoD could increase the enrollment fees, copayments, and deductibles that retirees pay to access TRICARE. Or it could exclude working-age retirees from participation in TRICARE Prime—the most costly plan for the government and the one with the lowest out-of-pocket costs for beneficiaries—while still allowing them to use Standard or Extra.

Each of these approaches has the potential to reduce spending for military health care, but each has drawbacks as well. CBO examined specific ways that the approaches

could be implemented and found that the last one—increasing beneficiaries' cost sharing—has by far the greatest likelihood of significantly reducing DoD's health care costs.

Improve Patients' Health by Better Managing Chronic Diseases

TRICARE has instituted several disease management programs. In principle, those programs could produce long-term savings even if they raised near-term costs. Most such programs have three components:

■ Educating patients about their condition and how to manage it themselves;

■ Actively monitoring patients' clinical symptoms and treatment plans; and

■ Coordinating care among all providers, including specialists, hospitals, and pharmacies.

However, although disease management programs have the potential to improve health outcomes, DoD's experience to date suggests that savings from such programs would probably be small.

DoD has sponsored three studies to evaluate the cost-effectiveness of its disease management programs—only one of which the department made available to CBO for review.[1] That study examined 57,000 participants in the first such program instituted by TRICARE, which was

---

1. DoD noted that the other two studies (which involved programs offered for the treatment of additional types of chronic illnesses) did not demonstrate net savings.

designed to manage treatment of three chronic conditions: asthma, congestive heart failure, and diabetes.[2] Over the two-year evaluation period, TRICARE beneficiaries with those diseases experienced fewer admissions for emergencies and inpatient care and incurred lower medical costs than those experienced by a control group of similar people. In addition, with a few exceptions, increased percentages of patients received appropriate medications and tests. The estimated overall savings across the program averaged $1.26 per $1.00 spent on disease management services. That is, the program cost an estimated $22.7 million to operate and yielded estimated gross savings of $28.5 million, a net savings of $5.8 million, or about 12 percent of what DoD otherwise would have spent on health care for those patients.[3]

For people suffering with asthma, the researchers estimated average annual medical savings (net of program costs) of $94 per patient. For patients with congestive heart failure, the net savings averaged $77 per person; and for diabetes patients, the net savings per person averaged $162. DoD estimated at the time that the populations of TRICARE patients suffering from asthma, congestive heart failure, and diabetes were 80,000, 11,000, and 225,000, respectively. To get an approximate estimate of the annual savings possible from expanding disease management programs, CBO multiplied the estimated net savings per person by half the eligible population identified by DoD in 2008 (for each of the three groups). CBO did not include the entire population because some people might have already entered disease management programs since then. Also, the original data included patients who were sicker than average (that is, identified as most likely to benefit from disease management programs). Thus, it is unlikely that the estimated

per-person savings would pertain to the entire population of individuals with those diseases.

Applying the annual per-patient rate to half of the populations with each disease studied suggests average annual savings of $23 million (in 2014 dollars) for all three diseases combined. Even if the entire population was included, savings would be less than $46 million per year—only 0.1 percent of total TRICARE costs. DoD has added several additional conditions to its disease management programs since 2008: depression, anxiety, and chronic pulmonary obstructive disease. If all three were considered, the expanded population could be as high as 600,000. But DoD reported to CBO that no net savings have been realized from the newer programs so far, so CBO did not estimate additional savings associated with those illnesses.

TRICARE's disease management programs did not include patients who were eligible for Medicare, so the groups being evaluated tended to be younger (and therefore healthier, even given their chronic conditions) than their counterparts in studies focusing on Medicare populations. Nevertheless, the results of the TRICARE programs—that is, no substantial savings—are similar to results for the Medicare program. Those studies have found that, when the fees paid to participating organizations were considered, most disease management and care coordination programs have not reduced Medicare spending.[4]

Administer the Military Health Care System More Effectively

To reduce health care spending, DoD could alter its operations without affecting patients directly. CBO explored the effects of two such approaches:

- *Educate military physicians in a less costly way.* This approach would expand the use of scholarships for the education of military health care professionals in civilian universities. In addition, the only federally operated medical school—DoD's Uniformed Services University of the Health Sciences—would be closed.

2.   The results of the evaluation are reported in two publications. See Wenya Yang and others, "Disease Management 360: A Scorecard Approach to Evaluating TRICARE's Programs for Asthma, Congestive Heart Failure, and Diabetes," *Medical Care*, vol. 48, no. 8 (August 2010), http://tinyurl.com/qgk5jwu; and Timothy M. Dall and others, "Outcomes and Lessons Learned From Evaluating TRICARE's Disease Management Programs," *American Journal of Managed Care*, vol. 16, no. 6 (June 2010), pp. 438–446, http://tinyurl.com/pltdfhc.

3.   Timothy M. Dall and others, "Outcomes and Lessons Learned From Evaluating TRICARE's Disease Management Programs," *American Journal of Managed Care*, vol. 16, no. 6 (June 2010), p. 441, http://tinyurl.com/pltdfhc. The authors note that the program costs reflected in their results excluded DoD's administrative costs for oversight and contract implementation.

4.   See Congressional Budget Office, *Lessons from Medicare's Demonstration Projects on Disease Management, Care Coordination, and Value-Based Payment* (January 2012), www.cbo.gov/publication/42860.

■ *Hire additional auditors.* Extra auditors would be hired to reduce waste, fraud, and abuse in military medicine.

Any savings realized by making such changes would have a small effect on a $50 billion program. Nor would changes in administrative procedures address one of the key drivers of DoD's increased health care spending: beneficiaries' greater use of health care services.

Educate Military Physicians in a Less Costly Way

DoD has two main programs to recruit doctors:

■ In any given year, between 60 percent and 80 percent of prospective physicians entering the military do so through the Health Professionals Scholarship Program, which covers tuition (in full) at civilian medical schools, expenses for books, and other fees, plus a stipend in return for a military service obligation. (The service obligation is one year of service for each year of scholarship, with a minimum of three years of service.)

■ Each year, new graduates from the USUHS account for 8 percent to 15 percent of military physicians. Medical students who enter USUHS are commissioned as officers and receive military pay and benefits. In addition, tuition, expenses for books, and other fees are covered in full, in exchange for a longer (seven-year) service commitment.

Researchers have estimated that the cost of putting a student through medical school at USUHS is about three times the cost of using the scholarship program.[5]

One approach to reducing spending for military medical education would be to close USUHS and expand the scholarship program. For example, the class of 2018 (that is, the class entering in September 2014) could become the final graduating class of USUHS. If that approach was adopted, other types of medical training currently provided at USUHS, such as the Graduate School of Nursing and the Postgraduate Dental College, would

also be provided at civilian academic institutions. Military-specific continuing education courses would be transferred to other institutions inside and outside of DoD.[6] The military personnel currently assigned to USUHS would be reassigned to other military medical functions.

About 165 physicians graduate from USUHS each year; total enrollment in the medical school is about 680.[7] In 2012, the operation and maintenance budget of USUHS was about $190 million, which funded 570 civilian staff and 227 civilian faculty members. In addition, there are about 380 military members of the faculty and staff, representing about another $35 million per year in spending for military personnel.

Closing USUHS and funding additional scholarships for physicians—which CBO estimates would reduce spending by as much as $150 million per year—would have a small effect on the DoD's overall budget. That is because USUHS is relatively small, and the savings derived from closing the school would be diminished by the need to fund additional scholarships and continuing medical education.

Hire Additional Auditors

Under this approach, DoD would add staff to TRICARE's Program Integrity Office to reduce health care fraud, which is seen as a substantial problem throughout the economy. The Federal Bureau of Investigation has estimated that fraudulent billing accounts for between 3 percent and 10 percent of health care expenditures nationwide, for example.[8] A recent study of waste in health care spending estimated the same range for fraud

---

5. The most recent study available to CBO estimated the four-year cost of putting a student through USUHS at $960,000, while the cost of using the scholarship program was estimated to be $317,000 over four years (in 2014 dollars). See Robert A. Levy, Eric W. Christensen, and Senanu Asamoah, *Raising the Bonus and Prospects for DoD's Attracting Fully Trained Medical Personnel,* CRM D0013237.A2 (CNA Corporation, February 2006).

6. DoD already partners with civilian medical schools and facilities for certain programs, offering, for example, an orthopedic doctoral degree through Baylor University and Brooke Army Medical Center.

7. USUHS also offers advanced degrees in biomedical science and public health to military personnel and federal civilian employees. Currently about 180 graduate students are enrolled. Tuition is free, and competitive stipends ranging from $27,000 to $32,000 per year are available. Civilian students incur no military service obligation. USUHS also offers advanced degrees in nursing and dentistry and nondegree medical education courses.

8. See Federal Bureau of Investigation, *Financial Crimes Report to the Public, Fiscal Years 2010–2011* (October 1, 2009–September 30, 2011), www.fbi.gov/stats-services/publications/financial-crimes-report-2010-2011/financial-crimes-report-2010-2011#Health.

and abuse in Medicare and Medicaid in 2011.[9] If 3 percent of the cost of purchased care in the DHP was the result of fraud, the cost to DoD of that fraud would have been about $450 million in 2013. However, CBO does not have the data necessary to estimate the prevalence of fraud in the TRICARE program.

TRICARE's Office of Program Integrity investigates allegations of improper payments to civilian contractors as well as medical identity theft and eligibility fraud. Cases of suspected fraud are forwarded to the Defense Criminal Investigative Service and other federal law enforcement agencies. Identifying and recovering stolen funds can require many years of investigation, so linking the financial investment in investigations with cost reductions can be challenging. Periodically, CBO has provided estimates of the effect of devoting additional resources to reducing waste, fraud, and abuse in other federal health care programs. In some recent estimates, CBO projected that every additional $1.00 that the government spent on those activities would yield $1.50 in reduced health care expenditures.[10] The estimated return of 1.5 to 1 is similar to previous estimates by the Centers for Medicare & Medicaid Services for funding increases proposed in the President's budget.

As of 2010, the TRICARE Program Integrity Office maintained an antifraud division with nine auditors (plus management and administrative support). Doubling the size of that office might increase DoD's discretionary spending (outlays subject to annual appropriation acts) by about $1.3 million each year. However, the additional staff might reduce outlays for TRICARE benefits by roughly $2 million per year (if DoD was able to achieve the same savings that other federal health care programs have achieved by reducing fraud).[11] Expanding the program substantially, say by increasing it tenfold, could result in additional savings, but that would still be only a tiny fraction of TRICARE spending. With such a large increase in funding, additional considerations would

apply. For example, there might be decreasing marginal returns for each additional auditor hired; thus, the potential $1.50 figure used above might be too high. Moreover, CBO's analysis suggests that the expanded benefits and the financial attractiveness of TRICARE outlined in Chapter 1 have driven the growth in health care spending to a much greater extent than has fraud.

Increase Cost Sharing for Retirees Who Use TRICARE

One way to reduce spending for military health care would be to increase—or in some cases introduce—cost sharing for certain TRICARE users. Among the ways to do that would be to increase enrollment fees (which are similar to the premiums civilians pay for their insurance), copayments, and deductibles for those users. In addition, DoD could prevent certain populations from enrolling in the most heavily subsidized plan but allow them to remain in the TRICARE components that have greater cost sharing.

Since TRICARE began, DoD has periodically proposed changing the program's cost-sharing structure as a way to reduce federal spending. Such proposals, which focused primarily on retirees, have been made as part of DoD's budget requests almost every year since 2007, including 2014. The Congress has not approved large increases in the enrollment fees, although it authorized an increase in Prime enrollment fees for military retirees from $230 per year to $260 for single coverage and from $460 to $520 for families, starting in fiscal year 2012.[12] Lawmakers also authorized a further 3.6 percent increase in the fees—to $269 for singles and $539 for families—effective in October 2012. Despite those changes, enrollment fees are still substantially below the amounts that most civilians pay for employment-based health insurance, as are

9. See Donald M. Berwick and Andrew D. Hackbarth, "Eliminating Waste in US Health Care," *Journal of the American Medical Association,* vol. 307, no. 14 (April 11, 2012), pp. 1513–1516.

10. See, for example, Congressional Budget Office, letter to the Honorable John A. Boehner regarding the estimated impact on the budget of the Budget Control Act of 2011 (July 27, 2011), pp. 3–4 and Table 2, www.cbo.gov/publication/41611. The estimated savings from the program integrity activities undertaken in one year are spread out over multiple years.

11. Although additional discretionary funding for this type of program might lead to budgetary savings (from reduced benefit payments), pursuant to scorekeeping guidelines established by the Congress, savings in mandatory spending cannot be credited to provisions that would change the amount appropriated for administrative or program management activities.

12. The higher fees went into effect on October 1, 2011, for new enrollees during fiscal year 2012 and on October 1, 2012, for all enrollees. In future years, DoD has the authority to raise enrollment fees for TRICARE Prime at the same rate that military retirement pay rises (that is, both increases are based on the percentage increase in the consumer price index).

copayments and deductibles, which have remained largely unchanged since 1995.

Shifting current cost-sharing arrangements so that beneficiaries pay a greater percentage of their health care costs would reduce DoD's spending significantly, CBO estimates, primarily by encouraging people to leave TRICARE in favor of other providers.[13] It would also encourage those who continued to participate in TRICARE to use fewer services.

In this report, CBO explores three specific options that would institute changes to TRICARE's current cost-sharing structure and lead to reduced federal spending for military health care.[14]

■ *Option 1* would increase the enrollment fees, copayments, and deductibles paid by working-age retirees who use TRICARE, beginning in 2015. Those increases would reduce TRICARE's outlays by $23 billion over the 10-year period spanning 2014 to 2023, CBO estimates. The reduction to the federal deficit would be smaller, however, because of changes in other federal accounts. Discretionary spending would increase by about $3 billion for the Veterans Health Administration and the Federal Employees Health Benefits (FEHB) program because some users would switch to those programs. Mandatory spending for retired members of the Coast Guard and commissioned officers of the Public Health Service and of the National Oceanic and Atmospheric Administration (NOAA) would decline, but some retirees would rely more heavily on certain other federal programs, such as Medicaid; the net effect is that mandatory spending would decline by about $0.3 billion over the 10-year period. Also, revenues would decrease by about $1.6 billion from this option because many retirees would increase their usage of employment-based health care plans, which would reduce taxable compensation. The net reduction in

the federal deficit would be about $18 billion, if lawmakers reduced total appropriations accordingly.

■ *Option 2* would prevent working-age retirees and their families from enrolling in TRICARE Prime but would allow them to continue to participate in Standard or Extra by paying a new annual enrollment fee. CBO estimates that this change, if implemented at the start of 2015, would reduce TRICARE's outlays by about $85 billion over the 2014–2023 period. That reduction in spending would be partially offset by an increase of $14 billion in discretionary outlays by the Veterans Health Administration and FEHB program over the 10-year period. Mandatory outlays would increase by about $0.5 billion, and revenues would fall by about $11 billion between 2014 and 2023. Overall, this option would reduce the federal deficit by about $60 billion over 10 years, if lawmakers reduced total appropriations accordingly.

■ *Option 3* would require Medicare-eligible beneficiaries enrolled in TRICARE for Life at the start of 2015 (or later) to pay a portion of the costs for their health care. Those out-of-pocket costs would be capped so that Medicare and TRICARE, in combination, would pay 100 percent of allowable costs beyond that cap. (The cap would be set at $3,025 in the first year of implementation.) CBO estimates that, under this option, federal outlays from the Medicare-Eligible Retiree Health Care Fund and for Medicare (and, therefore, the federal deficit) would be reduced by a total of $31 billion over the 2014–2023 period.

The estimated spending reductions realized by implementing these options would not necessarily be additive. For instance, savings could not be realized by raising the enrollment fees that military retirees pay to join TRICARE Prime (as in Option 1) if they were prevented from enrolling in Prime at all (as in Option 2). However, either Option 1 or Option 2 could be combined with Option 3.

These three options would exempt active-duty service members and their families from any changes. It has long been argued that those families should receive easy and low-cost access to health care so that family health issues and related financial burdens do not weigh on the minds of service members, especially those who are deployed overseas.

---

13. See Congressional Budget Office, *The Effects of Proposals to Increase Cost Sharing in TRICARE* (June 2009), www.cbo.gov/publication/41188, for a detailed discussion of the effects of inducing people to leave TRICARE and the reduced consumption of health care services among those who stay.

14. The estimates in this report can also be found (in less detail) in Congressional Budget Office, *Options for Reducing the Deficit: 2014 to 2023* (November 2013), p. 203 and pp. 236–238, www.cbo.gov/budget-options/2013/44687.

Effects of Increased Cost Sharing on Beneficiaries' Health

In the options that CBO examined, TRICARE's enrollment fees, copayments, and deductibles for military retirees would more closely match the cost-sharing arrangements seen in civilian plans. Economic studies regarding civilians have shown that increases in cost sharing reduce the amount of health care that people use, including both effective and less-effective services, but the resulting consequences for people's overall health vary. Among some segments of the population—the elderly, those with chronic conditions, and those with low incomes, for example—the prospect of higher out-of-pocket costs may cause people to cut back on preventive care or the appropriate use of pharmaceuticals, resulting in greater need for acute care services.[15] However, none of the published studies on spending and health outcomes have specifically examined TRICARE beneficiaries, so many of these findings may not apply to them. Most TRICARE beneficiaries are not elderly and tend to use more health care services than comparable civilians, so reduced utilization might simply bring their consumption of health care services more in line with that of the overall civilian population. If so, it would probably not have significant effects on people's health.[16] Moreover, under the cost-sharing options examined by CBO, the TRICARE fees, copayments, and deductibles would approach the average out-of-pocket costs required by civilian plans, although the low costs that retirees pay for prescription drugs would not change at all.[17] Military

retirees' health might not be affected if the higher costs fostered more disciplined use of medical resources and primarily discouraged the use of low-value health care.

Options 1 and 2 would affect younger military retirees, most of whom are between the ages of 40 and 64. Their younger age and the likelihood that they will continue to work after they retire from the military would lessen the risk of adverse health outcomes for those most affected by the options. Option 3, which would make the TRICARE for Life benefit less generous, would leave Medicare-eligible beneficiaries enrolled in Medicare Part B, and their out-of-pocket expenditures would be capped. Nevertheless, some patients could face adverse health outcomes if the higher costs caused them to delay seeking care. Slowing the implementation of the options, or allowing exceptions for older or sicker retirees or those with lower earnings, would reduce such risks but also would diminish the potential savings over the next 10 years.

Other Issues Related to Increased Cost Sharing

One argument in favor of requiring retired personnel to pay more is that military health care benefits (TRICARE coverage and care provided at military treatment facilities on a space-available basis) were originally intended to supplement benefits offered by civilian employers or by Medicare once service members retired; coverage under TRICARE was not meant to replace those benefits. A second such argument involves equity among service members. Only about 15 percent of enlisted personnel, and half of officers, serve the 20 years required to retire from the military.[18] Thus, most of the members who have served in Iraq and Afghanistan, for example, will not benefit from the low-cost health care provided to military retirees.

An argument against changing the current cost-sharing arrangements is that such changes could be considered unfair: Some current retirees made decisions about continuing their period of active-duty service with the understanding that they would receive subsidized medical care after retiring from the military. Significantly limiting TRICARE coverage for military retirees and their

---

15. For an overview of the literature, see Katherine Swartz, *Cost-Sharing: Effects on Spending and Outcomes*, Research Synthesis Report 20 (Robert Wood Johnson Foundation, December 2010), http://tinyurl.com/oyle4s8. See, also, Michael E. Chernew and Joseph P. Newhouse, "What Does a RAND Health Insurance Experiment Tell Us About the Impact of Patient Cost Sharing on Health Outcomes?" *American Journal of Managed Care* (July 15, 2008), http://tinyurl.com/hd46bqp; and Amitabh Chandra, Jonathan Gruber, and Robin McKnight, "Patient Cost-Sharing and Hospitalization Offsets in the Elderly," *American Economic Review* (March 2010), pp. 193–213, http://tinyurl.com/lwe936n.

16. Department of Defense, *Evaluation of the TRICARE Program—Access, Cost and Quality: Fiscal Year 2013 Report to Congress* (February 2013), pp. 67 and 72, http://go.usa.gov/jX9H.

17. Military retirees pay nothing if they fill their prescriptions at military treatment facilities. If they use TRICARE's mail-order option, a 90-day supply of generic prescription drugs is free, and if they go to a retail pharmacy, a 30-day supply of a generic drug is $5. Copayments for brand-name drugs are higher: $13 for a 90-day supply through mail-order and $17 for a 30-day supply through a retail pharmacy.

18. Congressional Budget Office, *Evaluating Military Compensation* (June 2007), p. 15, www.cbo.gov/publication/18788. Service members who are medically disabled may receive a disability retirement pension even if they served for fewer than 20 years. Members who leave the service before retiring may be eligible for health care from the Veterans Health Administration.

dependents would impose an unexpected financial cost on many of them. Relatedly, the anticipation of low out-of-pocket costs in the future may encourage older members to remain for an entire career, and the experience those longer-serving members provide would benefit the military.

Estimated Budgetary Effects of Cost-Sharing Options

The three options outlined here would reduce federal budget deficits by amounts ranging from roughly $20 billion to $60 billion over the next 10 years, CBO estimates, if total appropriations were reduced accordingly. Although this study focuses on DoD's health care spending, the estimates below include the effects on all seven branches of the uniformed services; most of the projected savings would accrue to DoD, however.

Option 1: Increase Medical Cost Sharing for Military Retirees Who Are Not Yet Eligible for Medicare.

Under this option, DoD would raise the enrollment fees, co-payments, and deductibles for younger military retirees—those who are not yet eligible for Medicare—who wished to use TRICARE. Beginning in 2015, beneficiaries with single coverage could enroll in TRICARE Prime by paying a $550 annual fee, and those with family coverage could enroll for a $1,100 annual fee. That family enrollment fee would be approximately equivalent to the $460 fee first instituted in 1995, after adjusting for the nationwide growth in health care spending per capita. Under this option, each medical visit to a Prime provider in the civilian network would entail a copayment of $30, which, again, is approximately equivalent to the amount that was established in 1995. Copayments for other health services, such as inpatient care, would be adjusted accordingly (to keep the relative costs the same). Retirees (or surviving spouses) who wanted single coverage in TRICARE Standard or Extra would face an annual deductible of $350; the annual deductible for families would be $700. Those increases would also be consistent with the nationwide growth in per capita health care spending since 1995. In addition—and for the first time—users of TRICARE Standard or Extra would be required to enroll and pay an annual enrollment fee of $50 for single coverage and $100 for family coverage. All of those new or increased fees, copayments, and deductibles would be indexed to reflect future growth nationwide in per capita spending for health care.

If TRICARE fees, copayments, and deductibles were modified as specified in this option, CBO estimates, outlays for the TRICARE program would be reduced, on net, by about $23 billion over the 2014–2023 period (see Table 2-1). But the effect on the federal deficit would be somewhat smaller because the option would cause some eligible retirees to switch to other federal health care programs, such as the Federal Employees Health Benefits program (if the person or his or her spouse was employed as a civilian by the federal government) or that offered by the Veterans Health Administration, both of which are funded through annual appropriations. Some $3 billion in additional outlays would be needed for those programs over the 2014–2023 period, CBO projects, so the net reduction in discretionary spending would be about $20 billion over that 10-year period.

At the same time, some low-income people would switch to Medicaid, which would increase mandatory spending. (Lawmakers generally determine mandatory spending by setting each program's parameters, such as eligibility rules and benefit formulas, rather than by appropriating specific amounts each year.) However, those increases in mandatory spending would be more than offset by reduced mandatory spending for retired members of the Coast Guard and commissioned officers of the Public Health Service and of NOAA, the net effect being that overall mandatory spending would fall by $0.3 billion over 10 years.[19]

The changes in TRICARE fees also would cause some working retirees to shift to health care plans sponsored by their employers in the private sector. Because employment-based health insurance premiums are not subject to federal income tax, the change would lead to a shift in overall compensation from taxable wages to nontaxable fringe benefits. CBO and the staff of the Joint Committee on Taxation (JCT) estimate that this shift would result in a reduction of $1.6 billion in federal revenues over 10 years.[20] Thus, the net reduction to the federal deficit from this option would be about $18 billion, if lawmakers reduced total appropriations accordingly.

---

19. Health care costs for retired uniformed members of the Coast Guard, NOAA, and the Public Health Service are paid from mandatory spending accounts, which do not require annual appropriations. By contrast, DoD pays for the health care of its working-age retirees out of its annual discretionary appropriation.

20. Of the estimated $1.6 billion reduction in revenues that would result from 2014 through 2023, about $450 million would come from Social Security payroll taxes and would be classified as off-budget.

Table 2-1.

Estimated Budgetary Impact of Option 1: Increase Medical Cost Sharing for Military Retirees Not Yet Eligible for Medicare

(Billions of dollars)

	2014	2015	2016	2017	2018	2019	2020	2021	2022	2023	Total, 2014- 2023
Changes in Discretionary Spending											
DoD and the Uniformed Services											
Budget authority	0	-1.1	-1.7	-2.4	-2.6	-2.8	-3.0	-3.3	-3.5	-3.8	-24.1
Outlays	0	-0.9	-1.5	-2.2	-2.5	-2.7	-2.9	-3.1	-3.4	-3.6	-22.7
Veterans Health Administration and FEHB Program											
Budget authority	0	0.1	0.2	0.3	0.4	0.4	0.4	0.4	0.5	0.5	3.2
Outlays	0	0.1	0.2	0.3	0.3	0.4	0.4	0.4	0.5	0.5	3.0
Net Impact on Discretionary Spending											
Budget authority	0	-1.0	-1.5	-2.0	-2.2	-2.4	-2.6	-2.8	-3.0	-3.3	-21.0
Outlays	0	-0.8	-1.3	-1.9	-2.1	-2.3	-2.5	-2.7	-2.9	-3.1	-19.7
Other Budgetary Effects											
Change in mandatory outlays[a]	0	*	*	*	*	*	*	*	*	*	-0.3
Change in revenues[b]	0	*	-0.1	-0.1	-0.2	-0.2	-0.2	-0.2	-0.2	-0.3	-1.6

Sources: Congressional Budget Office and the staff of the Joint Committee on Taxation.

Notes: This option would increase the enrollment fee for TRICARE Prime to $550 for individuals and $1,100 for families. It also would increase copayments for Prime. In addition, it would create an enrollment fee of $50 for individuals and $100 for families for TRICARE Standard and Extra and would increase the deductibles for individuals and families to $350 and $700, respectively. All fees and deductibles would increase each year at the nationwide rate of growth in per capita spending for health care. This estimate is based on the assumption that the change would become effective beginning in fiscal year 2015.

Budget authority is authority provided by law to enter into obligations that will result in outlays of federal funds. Outlays are payments made to liquidate obligations.

DoD = Department of Defense; FEHB = Federal Employees Health Benefits; * = between -$50 million and $50 million.

a. Mandatory spending would increase because some retirees would rely more heavily on certain mandatory federal programs, such as Medicaid (if they have low incomes) or the FEHB program (if they have retired from the federal civil service). However, mandatory spending for health care would decline for retirees associated with the Coast Guard, the Commissioned Officer Corps of the National Oceanic and Atmospheric Administration, and the uniformed corps of the Public Health Service. The combined effect is shown in the table.

b. Negative numbers represent reductions in outlays or budget authority or a loss of revenues. About 30 percent of the estimated loss of revenues for each year would come from Social Security payroll taxes and so would be classified as off-budget. A loss of revenue would result because many retirees would increase their usage of employment-based health care plans, which would reduce taxable compensation.

Option 2: Make Military Retirees Ineligible for TRICARE Prime; Allow Continued Use of Standard and Extra With an Annual Fee. This option would make working-age military retirees and their dependents ineligible for enrollment in TRICARE Prime, which is the TRICARE plan with the lowest out-of-pocket costs for beneficiaries (and the most costly plan for DoD). Beginning in 2015, military retirees and their dependents would be able to

enroll in TRICARE Standard or Extra during an annual open enrollment period or when a qualifying life event occurred (for example, a change in marital status). Enrollees would pay a monthly premium that would be set at 28 percent of the cost of providing benefits for that group. That premium would be updated annually on the basis of the average cost the group incurred in the previous year. In addition, the catastrophic cap (maximum

Table 2-2.

Estimated Budgetary Impact of Option 2: Make Military Retirees Ineligible for Enrollment in TRICARE Prime; Allow Continued Use of TRICARE Standard or Extra With an Annual Fee

(Billions of dollars)

	2014	2015	2016	2017	2018	2019	2020	2021	2022	2023	Total 2014- 2023
Changes in Discretionary Spending											
DoD and the Uniformed Services											
Budget Authority	0	-4.1	-6.5	-9.3	-9.9	-10.5	-11.2	-11.9	-12.7	-13.4	-89.6
Outlays	0	-3.2	-5.8	-8.5	-9.5	-10.2	-10.8	-11.5	-12.2	-13.0	-84.6
Veterans Health Administration and FEHB Program											
Budget Authority	0	0.3	0.8	1.5	1.6	1.7	1.9	2.0	2.1	2.2	14.2
Outlays	0	0.3	0.7	1.3	1.6	1.7	1.8	2.0	2.1	2.2	13.7
Net Impact on Discretionary Spending											
Budget authority	0	-3.7	-5.7	-7.8	-8.3	-8.8	-9.4	-9.9	-10.6	-11.2	-75.4
Outlays	0	-3.0	-5.1	-7.1	-7.9	-8.4	-9.0	-9.6	-10.2	-10.8	-71.0
Other Budgetary Effects											
Change in mandatory outlays[a]	0	*	*	*	0.1	0.1	0.1	0.1	0.1	0.1	0.5
Change in revenues[b]	0	-0.2	-0.6	-1.0	-1.2	-1.3	-1.4	-1.5	-1.6	-1.6	-10.5

Source: Congressional Budget Office and the staff of the Joint Committee on Taxation.

Notes: This option would make working-age military retirees and their dependents ineligible for TRICARE Prime. They would be allowed to enroll in TRICARE Standard or Extra but would have to pay an annual fee equal to 28 percent of the government's cost of providing care under that program. The Standard or Extra deductibles and catastrophic cap would also be allowed to increase at the nationwide rate of growth in per capita spending for health care. This estimate is based on the assumption that the change would become effective beginning in fiscal year 2015.

      Budget authority is authority provided by law to enter into obligations that will result in outlays of federal funds. Outlays are payments made to liquidate obligations.

      DoD = Department of Defense; FEHB = Federal Employees Health Benefits; * = between -$50 million and $50 million.

a. Mandatory spending would increase because some retirees would rely more heavily on certain mandatory federal programs, such as Medicaid (if they have low incomes) or the FEHB program (if they have retired from the federal civil service). However, mandatory spending for health care would decline for retirees associated with the Coast Guard, the Commissioned Officer Corps of the National Oceanic and Atmospheric Administration, and the uniformed corps of the Public Health Service. The combined effect is shown in the table.

b. Negative numbers represent reductions in outlays or budget authority or a loss of revenues. About 30 percent of the estimated loss of revenues for each year would come from Social Security payroll taxes and so would be classified as off-budget. A loss of revenue would result because many retirees would increase their usage of employment-based health care plans, which would reduce taxable compensation.

out-of-pocket expenses) for military retirees and their dependents would be raised from the current $3,000 per family to $7,500 per family, the level at which it was set before January 2002. That catastrophic cap would increase in future years, with changes indexed to nationwide growth in per capita health care spending. If those changes were implemented at the beginning of 2015, CBO estimates, discretionary outlays for TRICARE would be reduced by $85 billion between 2014 and 2023 (see Table 2-2).

Military retirees and their dependents would still have the option of seeking care at no cost on a space-available basis at military treatment facilities through TRICARE Standard. However, such patients would be considered lower priority than Prime enrollees when it came to getting appointments, and, as a result, they might have difficulty obtaining care on a space-available basis. For that reason, military retirees and their dependents would have an incentive to obtain other coverage rather than rely on military treatment facilities as their main source of medical care. About three-quarters of all retired military beneficiaries not yet eligible for Medicare have access to employment-based insurance through civilian jobs. However, CBO estimates that only about one-third currently opt to enroll in those plans. More would do so under this option. CBO and JCT estimate that federal tax revenues would drop by about $11 billion over the 2014–2023 period as those who signed up for employment-based health care plans in the private sector experienced a shift in compensation from taxable wages to nontaxable fringe benefits.[21]

If this option was implemented, some retirees and their dependents could be expected to switch to other federal programs for which they are eligible rather than transferring to a private civilian plan. As a result, discretionary outlays for the Veterans Health Administration and the FEHB program would increase by about $14 billion over the 2014–2023 period, CBO estimates.[22]

Mandatory spending would change as well, by a small amount. For example, low-income people might qualify for Medicaid or for subsidies provided through the new insurance exchanges established in accordance with the Affordable Care Act.[23] Mandatory spending also would increase for people who retire from a second career as a civilian in the federal government if they rely on the FEHB program instead of TRICARE. But the higher

---

21. About $3 billion of the $11 billion would be classified as off-budget.

22. Only military retirees (or their spouses) who were employed by the federal government as civilians would qualify for the FEHB program.

23. Currently, TRICARE beneficiaries are not eligible for subsidies through the insurance exchanges. This option would raise the enrollment fee for Standard and Extra to a sufficiently high amount that some lower-income families would find themselves needing to pay a family enrollment fee of about $3,000 yet not qualifying for subsidies on the civilian insurance exchanges. CBO assumed, therefore, that DoD would reduce the TRICARE fee for those who could demonstrate sufficiently low household income, and adjusted the estimate accordingly.

TRICARE fees would reduce health care spending by members of the Coast Guard and the commissioned corps of the Public Health Service and of NOAA, which are paid from mandatory appropriations.

All told, the net reduction in the federal deficit from adopting Option 2 would be about $60 billion, if lawmakers reduced total appropriations accordingly. Compared with Option 1, the effects of Option 2 on federal spending would be substantially larger because more TRICARE Prime users would be affected. Under Option 1, CBO estimates, higher out-of-pocket costs would cause about 200,000 beneficiaries to leave Prime. Option 2, however, would affect all retirees and their families who currently participate in Prime—about 1.6 million people—because they would be automatically disenrolled if the option was implemented.

Option 3: Introduce Minimum Out-of-Pocket Requirements for TRICARE for Life. This option would introduce minimum out-of-pocket requirements for beneficiaries who use TFL. Under this option, starting in 2015, TFL would not cover any of the first $550 of an enrollee's cost-sharing payments under Medicare and would cover only 50 percent of the next $4,950 in such payments. (Because all further cost sharing would be covered by TFL, enrollees would not be obliged to pay more than $3,025 in cost sharing in that year.)[24] Those dollar limits would be indexed to growth in average per capita Medicare costs (excluding Part D) for later years. This option reflects the assumption that DoD would collect payments from TFL beneficiaries seeking care from military treatment facilities that would be roughly comparable to the charges incurred at civilian facilities; those charges would reduce users' incentives to switch to military treatment facilities to avoid the out-of-pocket costs of using civilian facilities.

This policy change would affect the MERHCF in two ways. First, payments *from* the fund would be reduced. Because higher out-of-pocket costs would lead current Medicare-eligible beneficiaries to use fewer medical services, this option would reduce both Medicare spending and mandatory outlays from the MERHCF—the

---

24. The calculation is $550 + (0.5 \times \$4,950) = \$3,025$.

Table 2-3.

Estimated Budgetary Impact of Option 3: Introduce Minimum Out-of-Pocket Requirements Under TRICARE for Life

(Billions of dollars)

	2014	2015	2016	2017	2018	2019	2020	2021	2022	2023	2014-2023
Change in Mandatory Outlays											
MERHCF	0	-1.4	-2.0	-2.2	-2.4	-2.6	-2.7	-2.8	-3.0	-3.2	-22.0
Medicare	0	-0.2	-0.5	-0.9	-1.0	-1.1	-1.1	-1.2	-1.3	-1.3	-8.6
Total	**0**	**-1.6**	**-2.5**	**-3.1**	**-3.4**	**-3.6**	**-3.8**	**-4.0**	**-4.3**	**-4.5**	**-30.7**
Memorandum:											
Change in Discretionary											
Accrual Payments to the MERHCF[a]											
Budget Authority	0	-1.6	-1.7	-1.8	-1.9	-2.0	-2.2	-2.3	-2.4	-2.5	-18.4

Source: Congressional Budget Office.

Notes: This option is based on the assumption that TRICARE would not cover any of the first $550 of an enrollee's cost-sharing payments under Medicare and would cover only 50 percent of the next $4,950 in payments each year.

CBO's estimate is based on the assumption that the changes would become effective beginning in fiscal year 2015.

Budget authority is authority provided by law to enter into obligations that will result in outlays of federal funds. Outlays are payments made to liquidate obligations.

MERHCF = Medicare-Eligible Retiree Health Care Fund.

a. This option would reduce the Department of Defense's discretionary accrual payments to the MERHCF. However, those payments are recorded as intragovernmental transactions and would have no net impact on the deficit.

payments that the fund makes to reimburse TRICARE providers and to pay military treatment facilities for care delivered to Medicare-eligible retirees. As a result, CBO estimates, this option would reduce the amount of federal mandatory spending devoted to TFL beneficiaries and, therefore, the federal deficit by $31 billion through 2023 (see Table 2-3).

Second, payments *to* the MERHCF would be reduced as well. CBO estimates that DoD would be able to reduce its cumulative accrual payments to the MERHCF by about $18 billion over the 2014–2023 period. Although DoD would require less discretionary funding, payments to the MERHCF are intragovernmental transfers and therefore have no effect on the federal deficit. CBO therefore did not include reductions in accrual payments when calculating the effects on the federal deficit.

Appendix:
Cost Sharing in TRICARE

The fees, copayments, and deductibles that TRICARE users face depend on several factors: whether the beneficiary is serving on active duty, is a family member or surviving spouse of an active-duty service member, or is retired from the military. Other considerations are the type of TRICARE plan the beneficiary qualifies for and uses—Prime, Standard, or Extra—and whether the individual receives care in a military treatment facility or from a civilian provider.

This appendix provides an overview of the various fees that TRICARE users pay. The accompanying tables provide a more detailed breakdown of those costs.

■ Active-duty members and their families who use Prime pay no out-of-pocket costs (see Table A-1). Family members can use Standard or Extra, which allow more choice of providers but require a deductible and some cost-sharing payments.

■ Retirees and their families who are not yet eligible for Medicare (sometimes called working-age retirees) pay nothing if they rely on military facilities for their care. If they choose to use civilian providers within the Prime network, they face lower costs than those who rely on the Extra network or pay Standard fee-for-service charges (see Table A-2 on page 35). They pay a larger share of costs than family members of people on active duty.

■ Retired members and their families who are eligible for Medicare can join the TRICARE for Life program. Enrolling in that program is free but only those who have enrolled in Medicare Part B can participate. Medicare Part B premiums ranged between $1,260 and $4,030 in 2013, depending on the person's income and tax-filing status (see Table A-3 on page 36).

Table A-1.

Cost Sharing Under TRICARE for Active-Duty Service Members and Their Families, 2013

	TRICARE Prime[a]	TRICARE Extra[b]	TRICARE Standard
Annual Enrollment Fee	0	0	0
Annual Deductible	0	$50 single/$100 family for E-4 and below; $150 single/$300 family for E-5 and above	$50 single/$100 family for E-4 and below; $150 single/$300 family for E-5 and above
Outpatient Visit[c]	0	15 percent of negotiated charge	20 percent of allowed charges for covered service
Emergency Services[c]	0	15 percent of negotiated charge	20 percent of allowed charges for covered service
Mental Health Visit[c]	0	15 percent of negotiated charge	20 percent of allowed charges for covered service
Inpatient Hospitalization[c]	0	$17 per day ($25 minimum charge)	$17 per day ($25 minimum charge)
Catastrophic Cap[d]	$1,000	$1,000	$1,000

Source: Congressional Budget Office based on information from the Department of Defense.

Note: The military's TRICARE program provides health care to uniformed and retired service members and their dependents and survivors through an integrated system of military and civilian facilities and providers. The program comprises several health plans, the largest of which are TRICARE Prime, which operates similarly to a civilian health maintenance organization, and TRICARE Extra and Standard, two fee-for-service plans differentiated by beneficiaries' use of network versus nonnetwork providers.

a.   Active-duty personnel must use TRICARE Prime. Their family members can choose among Prime, Extra, and Standard. Users of Prime receive priority when making appointments in military facilities. Family members enrolled in Prime can see specialty providers without a referral under a "point-of-service" (POS) option. The POS option has a $300/$600 deductible and 50 percent cost share.

b.   Extra requires the use of a preferred provider network. Users who seek treatment outside of the network receive the Standard benefit.

c.   Charges apply to civilian providers only. Visits to or treatments by military providers involve no costs to TRICARE beneficiaries, although minimal charges may apply for inpatient services.

d.   The catastrophic cap is the annual maximum a family has to pay for TRICARE-covered services.

Table A-2.

Cost Sharing Under TRICARE for Working-Age Retirees and Their Families, 2013

	TRICARE Prime[a]	TRICARE Extra[b]	TRICARE Standard
Annual Enrollment	$269 single/$539 family	0	0
Annual Deductible	0	$150 single/$300 family	$150 single/$300 family
Outpatient Visit[c]	$12	20 percent of negotiated charge	25 percent of allowed charges
Emergency Services[c]	$30	20 percent of negotiated charge	25 percent of allowed charges
Mental Health Visit[c]	$25 individual/$17 group	20 percent of negotiated charge	25 percent of allowed charges
Inpatient Hospitalization[c]	$11 per day ($25 minimum)	In network: $250 per day or 25 percent for hospital services (whichever is less) plus 20 percent for separately billed professional charges	$698 per day or 25 percent of institutional services (whichever is less) plus 25 percent for separately billed professional charges
Catastrophic Cap[d]	$3,000	$3,000	$3,000

Source: Congressional Budget Office based on information from the Department of Defense.

Note: The military's TRICARE program provides health care to uniformed and retired service members and their dependents and survivors through an integrated system of military and civilian facilities and providers. The program comprises several health plans, the largest of which are TRICARE Prime, which operates similarly to a civilian health maintenance organization, and TRICARE Extra and Standard, two fee-for-service plans differentiated by beneficiaries' use of network versus nonnetwork providers.

a. Users of TRICARE Prime receive priority when making appointments in military facilities. Prime enrollees can see specialty providers without a referral under a "point-of-service" (POS) option. The POS option has a $300/$600 deductible and 50 percent cost share.

b. Extra requires the use of a preferred provider network. Users who seek treatment outside of the network receive the Standard benefit.

c. Charges apply to civilian providers only. Visits to or treatments by military providers involve no costs to TRICARE beneficiaries, although minimal charges may apply for inpatient services.

d. The catastrophic cap is the annual maximum a family has to pay for TRICARE-covered services.

Table A-3.

Medicare Part B Premiums for Individuals in 2013, by Tax-Filing Status and Income

Tax-Filing Status and Modified Adjusted Gross Income	Monthly Part B Premium (Dollars)	Annual Part B Premium (Dollars)
Individual with income less than or equal to $85,000 or married filing jointly with income less than or equal to $170,000	104.90	1,258.80
Individual with income greater than $85,000 but less than or equal to $107,000 or married filing jointly with income exceeding $170,000 but less than or equal to $214,000	146.90	1,762.80
Individual with income greater than $107,000 but less than or equal to $160,000 or married filing jointly with income greater than $214,000 but less than or equal to $320,000	209.80	2,517.60
Individual with income greater than $160,000 but less than or equal to $214,000 or married filing jointly with income more than $320,000 but less than or equal to $428,000	272.70	3,272.40
Individual with income greater than $214,000 or married filing jointly with income greater than $428,000	335.70	4,028.40

Source: Centers for Medicare & Medicaid Services.

Notes: The income measure is modified adjusted gross income in 2011 as defined by the Internal Revenue Service.

Medicare Part B covers outpatient health care. Premiums are the same for military and civilian retirees.

Each enrollee faces a $147 annual deductible.

List of Tables and Figures

Tables

Figures

About This Document

This Congressional Budget Office (CBO) report was prepared at the request of the Chairman of the House Committee on the Budget. In keeping with CBO's mandate to provide objective, impartial analysis, the report makes no recommendations.

Carla Tighe Murray of CBO's National Security Division prepared the report with guidance from David E. Mosher and Matthew S. Goldberg. Jean Hearne, Sarah Jennings, Bernard Kempinski, Sarah Masi, Julia Mitchell, and Matthew Schmit of CBO contributed to the report, as did the staff of the Joint Committee on Taxation.

Julie Somers, formerly of CBO's Health, Retirement, and Long-Term Analysis Division, C. Vance Gordon of the Institute of Defense Analyses, and Lewis G. Lee (retired Sergeant Major of the Marine Corps) of the CNA Corporation provided thoughtful reviews and helpful comments. The assistance of external reviewers implies no responsibility for the final product, which rests solely with CBO.

Loretta Lettner edited the report, and Jeanine Rees and Maureen Costantino prepared it for publication. An electronic version is available on CBO's website (www.cbo.gov/publication/44993).

Douglas W. Elmendorf
Director

January 2014